Pediatric Genetics and Inborn Errors of Metabolism

T0178055

Christine M. Houser

Pediatric Genetics and Inborn Errors of Metabolism

A Practically Painless Review

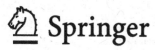 Springer

Christine M. Houser
Department of Emergency Medicine
Erasmus Medical Center
Rotterdam, The Netherlands

ISBN 978-1-4939-0580-5   ISBN 978-1-4939-0581-2 (eBook)
DOI 10.1007/978-1-4939-0581-2
Springer New York Heidelberg Dordrecht London

Library of Congress Control Number: 2014934567

Printed on acid-free paper

Springer is part of Springer Science+Business Media (www.springer.com)

To my parents Martin and Cathy who made this journey possible, to Patrick who travels it with me, and to my wonderful children Tristan, Skyler, Isabelle, Castiel, and Sunderland who have patiently waited during its writing – and are also the most special of all possible reminders for why pediatric medicine is so important.

Important Notice

Medical knowledge and the accepted standards of care change frequently. Conflicts are also found regularly in the information provided by various recognized sources in the medical field. Every effort has been made to ensure that the information contained in this publication is as up to date and accurate as possible. However, the parties involved in the publication of this book and its component parts, including the author, the content reviewers, and the publisher, do not guarantee that the information provided is in every case complete, accurate, or representative of the entire body of knowledge for a topic. We recommend that all readers review the current academic medical literature for any decisions regarding patient care.

Preface

Keeping all of the relevant information at your fingertips in a field as broad as pediatrics is both an important task and quite a lot to manage. Add to that the busy schedule most physicians and physicians-to-be carry of a practice or medical studies, family life, and sundry other personal and professional obligations, and it can be daunting. Whether you would like to keep your knowledge base up to date for your practice, are preparing for the general pediatric board examination or recertification, or are just doing your best to be well prepared for a ward rotation, *Pediatric Genetics and Inborn Errors of Metabolism* can be an invaluable asset.

This book brings together the information from several major pediatric board review study guides, and more review conferences than any one physician would ever have time to personally attend, so that you can review it at your own pace. It's important, especially if there isn't a lot of uninterrupted study time available, to find materials that make the study process as efficient and flexible as possible. What makes this book additionally unusual among medical study guides is its design using "bite-sized" chunks of information that can be quickly read and processed. Most information is presented in a question-and-answer (Q&A) format that improves attention and focus and ultimately learning. Critically important for most in medicine, it also enhances the speed with which the information can be learned.

Because the majority of information is in Q&A format, it is also much easier to use the information in a few minutes of downtime at the hospital or the office. You don't need to get deeply into the material to understand what you are reading. Each question and answer is brief – not paragraphs long as is often the case in medical review books – which means that the material can be moved through rapidly, keeping the focus on the most critical information.

At the same time, the items have been written to ensure that they contain the necessary information. Very often, information provided in review books raises as many questions as it answers. This interferes with the study process, because the learner either has to look up the additional information (time loss and hassle) or skip the information entirely – which means not really understanding and learning it. This book keeps answers self-contained, meaning that any needed information is provided either directly in the answer or immediately following it – all without lengthy text.

To provide additional study options, questions and answers are arranged in a simple two-column design, making it possible to easily cover one side and quiz yourself, or use the book for quizzing in pairs or study groups.

For a few especially challenging topics, or for the occasional topic that is better presented in a regular text style, a text section has been provided. These sections precede the larger Q&A section for that topic (so, for example, genetics text sections will precede the Q&A section for genetics). It is important to note that when text sections are present, they are not intended as an overview or an introduction to the Q&A section. They are stand-alone topics simply found to be more usefully presented as clearly written and relatively brief text sections.

The materials utilized in *Practically Painless Pediatrics* have been tested by residents and attendings preparing for the general pediatric board examination, or the recertification examination, to ensure that both the approach and content are on target. All content has also been reviewed by attending and specialist pediatricians to ensure its quality and understandability.

If you are using these materials to prepare for an exam, this can be a great opportunity to thoroughly review the many areas involved in pediatric practice and to consolidate and refresh the knowledge developed through the years so far. *Practically Painless Pediatrics* is available to cover the breadth of the topics included in the general pediatric board examination.

The formats and style in which materials are presented in *Practically Painless Pediatrics* utilize the knowledge gained about learning and memory processes over many years of research into cognitive processing. All of us involved in the process of creating it sincerely hope that you will find the study process a bit less onerous with this format and that it becomes at least at times an exciting adventure to refresh or build your knowledge.

Brief Guidance Regarding the Use of the Book

Items which appear in **bold** indicate topics known to be frequent board examination content. On occasion, an item's content is known to be very specific to previous board questions. In that case, the item will have "popular exam item" beneath it.

At times, you will encounter a Q&A item that covers the same content as a previous item. These items are worded differently and often require you to process the information in a somewhat different way compared to the previous version. This variation in the way questions from particularly challenging or important content areas are asked is not an error or an oversight. It is simply a way to easily and automatically practice the information again. These occasional repeat items are designed to increase the probability that the reader will be able to retrieve the information when it is needed – regardless of how the vignette is presented on the exam or how the patient presents in a clinical setting.

Occasionally, a brand name for a medication or a piece of medical equipment is included in the materials. These are indicated with the trademark symbol (®) and are not meant to indicate an endorsement of, or recommendation to use, that brand name product. Brand names are occasionally included only to make processing of the study items easier, in cases in which the brand name is significantly more recognizable to most physicians than the generic name would be.

The specific word choice used in the text may at times seem informal to the reader and occasionally a bit irreverent. Please rest assured that no disrespect is intended to anyone or any discipline, in any case. The mnemonics or comments provided are only intended to make the material more memorable. The informal wording is often easier to process than the rather complex or unusual wording many of us in the medical field have become accustomed to. That is why rather straightforward wording is sometimes used, even though it may at first seem unsophisticated.

Similarly, visual space is provided on the page, so that the material is not closely crowded together. This improves the ease of using the material for self- or group quizzing and minimizes the time potentially wasted identifying which answers belong to which questions.

The reader is encouraged to use the extra space surrounding items to make notes or add comments for himself or herself. Further, the Q&A format is particularly well suited to mark difficult or important items for later review and quizzing. If you are utilizing the book for exam preparation, please consider making a system in advance to indicate which items you'd like to return to, which items have already been repeatedly reviewed, and which items do not require further review. This not only makes the study process more efficient and less frustrating, but it can also offer a handy way to know which items are most important for last-minute review – frequently a very difficult "triage" task as the examination time approaches.

Finally, consider switching back and forth between topics under review to improve processing of new items. Trying to learn and remember many information items on similar topics is often more difficult than breaking the information into chunks by periodically switching to a different topic.

Ultimately, the most important aspect of learning the material needed for board and ward examinations is what we as physicians can bring to our patients – and the amazing gift that patients entrust to us in letting us take an active part in their health. With that focus in mind, the task at hand is not substantially different from what each examination candidate has already done successfully in medical school and in patient care. Keeping that uppermost in our minds, board examination studying should be both a bit less anxiety provoking and a bit more palatable. Seize the opportunity, and happy studying to all!

Rotterdam, The Netherlands   Christine M. Houser

About the Author

Dr. Houser completed her medical degree at the Johns Hopkins University School of Medicine, after spending 4 years in graduate training and research in cognitive neuropsychology at George Washington University and the National Institutes of Health (NIH). Her Master of Philosophy degree work focused on the processes involved in learning and memory, and during this time she was a four-time recipient of training awards from the NIH. Dr. Houser's dual interests in cognition and medicine led her naturally toward teaching and "translational cognitive science" – finding ways to apply the many years of cognitive research findings about learning and memory to how physicians and physicians-in-training might more easily learn and recall the vast quantities of information required for medical studies and practice.

Content Reviewers

For Genetics and Inborn Errors of Metabolism Topics

Saumya Shekhar Jamuar, MBBS, MRCPCH
Clinical Fellow, Division of Genetics and Metabolism
Boston Children's Hospital
Harvard Medical School Genetics Training Program
Boston, MA, USA

Vidhu Thaker, MD
Fellow, Pediatric Endocrinology
Boston Children's Hospital
Harvard University
Boston, MA, USA

Contents

Chapter 1
Genetic Concepts and Terminology

Chromosomal Conundrums: The Wacky World of Chromosomes That Want To Be Different

The basics: What are chromosomes supposed to do?

Chromosomes allow the cell to pass on genetic material in one of the two ways – mitosis and meiosis.

Mitosis is regular cell division. It creates more cells of the same differentiated type (for example, when gut or skin basal layer cells divide to produce more epithelial cells for the body).

Meiosis is limited to the "germ cells" or cells that will later produce gametes. "Gametes" is the general term for egg or sperm cells.

Meiosis has two stages, creatively named meiosis I and II.

Before meiosis I begins, the cell duplicates the 23 pairs of chromosomes it normally has, so that there is twice the usual amount of DNA/chromosomes in the cell.

(Remember that the 46 chromosomes normally present in human cells are actually *two sets* of 23 chromosomes. The germ cell from each parent usually contributes one member of each chromosome pair.)

In meiosis I, the doubled sets of chromosomes come together in the middle of the cell. *They have the opportunity at that point (during metaphase, specifically, when they are lined up) to "trade" some of their DNA between adjacent chromosomes. This is a normal process, meant to increase genetic diversity. The process is referred to as "recombination."*

C.M. Houser, *Pediatric Genetics and Inborn Errors of Metabolism:*
A Practically Painless Review, DOI 10.1007/978-1-4939-0581-2_1,
© Springer Science+Business Media New York 2014

After metaphase, the doubled sets of chromosomes split, so that a complete set can go to each of the two daughter cells.

In meiosis II, the homologous chromosomes (chromosomes with the same overall structure, although not necessarily the same base-pair sequence) separate and go to two different daughter cells. This produces the "haploid" germ cells with only 23 chromosomes, rather than 23 *pairs* of chromosomes.

(Note: The process described most accurately reflects what happens in male meiosis. The female process is the same in spirit, but not as many gametes are produced – because some of the chromosome sets produced just condense, rather than forming viable gamete cells.)

How do we know what chromosomes a person has?

Chromosomes are normally viewed microscopically by catching a cell in the act of cell division (mitosis). The chromosomes are visible to the microscopically aided eye when they are in either metaphase or prophase of the cell cycle.

The visual display of the chromosomes is, technically, the "karyotype."

Lymphocytes are the cell group most often used for karyotype analysis, because they are easy to obtain and they divide regularly. Skin fibroblasts are also used frequently. Any cell that divides, though, could be used.

What are autosomes?

Autosomes are the chromosomes that <u>don't</u> have to do with the gender of the individual. There are 22 "autosomal" chromosomes.

Who decided how the chromosomes should be numbered?

The autosomal chromosomes are numbered according to size from biggest to smallest (#1 is biggest).

The sex chromosomes, as you know, are simply labeled X or Y.

What is the correct way to write or describe a particular karyotype?

If you need to describe a karyotype, the correct nomenclature is as follows:

Part 1 – List the *number* of chromosomes (including the sex chromosomes).
Part 2 – List the *sex chromosome composition*.
Part 3 – List any *abnormalities*, such as deletions or translocations.

Examples:

46 XY	Normal male
46 XY, 5p-	5p- deletion (male)
47 XX, +21	Trisomy 21 (female)
45 XO	Turner's syndrome (one X sex chromosome)
45 XX, t(13q14q)	Robertsonian translocation of 13q and 14q

My mother told me to mind my p's and q's, but why do I keep seeing them in genetic analyses?

When describing a single chromosome, "p" refers to the short arm (p is for "petite"). "q" refers to the long arm of the chromosome (simply because that is the letter that follows "p" in the alphabet).

What does "chromosomal banding" mean?

"Bands" refer to the dark and light areas along the arms of the chromosomes. These areas can be seen when the cell is preparing to divide, because the genetic material is organized in a way that is easier to see than usual.

In addition to the chromosome's number, chromosomes are also referred to by their shape. They all look like X's to me. What is that about?

Chromosomes can be described according to the location of the centromere (the little belt-like thing holding the two homologous chromosomes together).

Belt in the center – If the centromere is exactly in the center, the chromosome is "metacentric."

Belt a little off-center – If the centromere is close to the center of the chromosome, but is just a little off toward one end, it is "submetacentric."

Belt is way off – Like wearing a belt around your neck to a funky club! – The final possibility is that the centromere is far from center, with just two little nubbins of genetic material on the end closest to the centromere. Chromosomes with this design are called "acrocentric."

Which phase of cell division gives the best visualization of chromosomes?

Prophase is the best possible portion of the cell cycle for viewing the chromosomes. They are longer and "less condensed" during prophase, compared to the other phases in which the chromosomes are visible. This means that more bands can be seen on the chromosome in prophase than at any other point in the cycle. Approximately 1,000 bands (or twice as many as in metaphase) can be seen.

Which phase of cell division is most often used to visualize the chromosomes?

Metaphase – not prophase! About 500 bands can be seen.

When would you want to examine both lymphocytes and skin fibroblasts for the patient's karyotype?

If mosaicism is suspected. It is possible that some of the body's cells have a different karyotype than the others.

If a cell is referred to as "aneuploid," what does that mean?

It has an incorrect number of chromosomes.

What is a "euploid" cell?

A cell that has _any multiple_ of the correct number of chromosomes, which is 23. This means that a cell with just 23 chromosomes is euploid, as is a cell with 46 chromosomes. A cell with 69 chromosomes is also, strangely enough, a euploid.

What are the special words to indicate that a cell is euploid but has an unusual multiple of 23 chromosomes?

Haploid – 23 chromosomes only
Polyploid – A multiple of 23 greater than 46 (such as 69)

What effect does it have on humans if they are missing an autosomal chromosome?

Missing an autosome is incompatible with life – except in two situations.

1. If the individual is mosaic, there may still be significant numbers of functional cells.
2. If the monosomy is partial, rather than complete, only a portion of the chromosome is missing. Sometimes these individuals survive.

What effect does it have on humans if they have extra autosomal chromosomes?

Most of the time, it is incompatible with life. Trisomy 21 is best tolerated, but even in trisomy 21, half of all conceptions spontaneously abort.

The only trisomies that can produce live-born infants are 13 (Patau), 18 (Edwards), and 21 (Down's).

How do cells make errors and end up with the wrong number of chromosomes?

One way is "nondisjunction." This means that when the chromosomes were supposed to separate during meiosis, one pair didn't. One daughter cell therefore ended up with an extra copy of one of the chromosomes. (This also means that another one of the daughter cells in the process will be short a chromosome.)

Anaphase lag, on the other hand, is when one of the chromosomes gets "lost" after separation. In this situation, separation of the daughter cell chromosomes and cell membranes occurs correctly, but one of the chromosomes just doesn't move fast enough to make it into the new cell. (It ends up outside the cell and is broken down.)

How common are chromosomal abnormalities in live-born babies?

Relatively common – about 0.4 % (very subtle abnormalities of genetic sequences are even more common).

How important are genetic disorders to the healthcare of children?

Pretty important.

Genetic disorders are frequent contributors to the need for hospital admissions at children's hospitals (about 40 % of children's hospital admissions are related to genetic disorders).

Genetic disorders are also a common cause of mortality in children, with 11 % of pediatric deaths related to underlying genetic disorders.

We've discussed extra chromosomes, missing chromosomes, and missing significant chunks of chromosomes (partial monosomy). There must be smaller errors in chromosomes that can also cause problems, aren't there?

Yes – there are a variety. They are grouped into the general categories of deletions, microdeletions, inversions, and translocations.

Deletion – The most straightforward is a deletion, in which a small part of a chromosome is missing. Not so much is missing that the chromosome is grossly smaller than usual, but the change in the banding pattern is visible in karyotype preparations.

Deletions are most likely to occur near the end of the chromosome (also known as the telomere). Deletions can be "simple" (part of the chromosome is missing) or "deletion with duplication" meaning that another chromosome segment was copied and put in place of the deleted material.

Small deletions are a common cause of mild mental retardation with associated mild congenital anomalies.

Common deletion syndromes include Cri du chat and Wolf–Hirschhorn (Greek helmet facies) syndromes.

Microdeletions – Microdeletion is just what it sounds like – a very small deletion of just a few genes. Microdeletions are clinically detectable by a typical phenotype or can sometimes be seen by inspection of a prometaphase preparation. (Sometimes, the deletion is too small to be microscopically detectable at all.)

Well-known syndromes that result from microdeletions include Angelman syndrome (happy puppet) and Prader–Willi and DiGeorge syndrome.

Inversions – Inversions are also what they sound like. Part of a chromosome flip-flops its direction on the chromosome. Although some of the genome is backwards after an inversion, the person who has it usually does not have any problems due to the inversion. This is because the amount of genetic material lost is usually quite small.

Although people with inversions are usually phenotypically normal, they are at increased risk for having abnormal gametes. This may seem strange, given that they don't have any trouble from the inversion themselves. The reason problems occur with the gametes is that the chromosomes have difficulty pairing up in meiosis. After an inversion occurs, the chromosomes that should be paired are no longer completely homologous. This means that they may not pair properly in metaphase. Improper pairing can cause the cell to delete or duplicate genetic material in an effort to fix the problem. The failure to pair properly, along with deletion or duplication of genes, leads to an abnormal gamete.

Inversions are quite common – 1 per 100 individuals has one.

Inversions are often designated as "pericentric" and "paracentric." This probably sounds like a boring and tedious distinction, but read on. *Sometimes you are expected to know which is which just by seeing a diagram of the abnormal chromosome beside a normal chromosome.*

Pericentric means that the inversion involved the centromere. In other words, the centromere flipped, also. A pericentric inversion is easy to recognize, because the centromere is in a different location after the flip occurs.

In a paracentric inversion, only chromosome arm material flip-flops. The centromere remains in its usual position. (*Mnemonic: "P__ara__" is in the __arm__ – PE__ri__ includes centromE__rE__.*)

Translocations – Translocation involves transfer of genetic material to a new chromosome location.

How is translocation different from recombination?

In translocation, genetic material is moved between nonhomologous chromosomes. In recombination, the exchange is between homologous chromosomes and results in increased diversity but no dysfunction.

Are there different types of translocations?

Yes. There are two general categories – reciprocal and Robertsonian.

Reciprocal means that two segments switched sites (traded) between different, non-homologous chromosomes. Very little genetic material is lost, if any. The material has just "moved" to a new residence on the genome.

Robertsonian translocation can only occur between two chromosomes that are acrocentric. (Acrocentric, remember, means that the centromere is situated very near to one end of the chromosome.) Bizarrely enough, the long arms of two *different* chromosomes fuse to make *a single* new chromosome. The short ends of the chromosome (the part that looks like Mickey Mouse ears at the top) are broken down by the cell. This means that the resulting person has 45 autosomes, rather than the usual 46.

Reciprocal translation doesn't seem so bad, since the material is just relocated. Do people with reciprocal translocations usually have problems due to the translocation?

No. They often have difficulty with miscarriages, though, due to gametes with abnormal amounts of genetic material.

(Remember that each chromosome has a paired homologue. Only one of the homologues participates in the translocation with some other chromosome homologue. This means that there is a normal and abnormal chromosome in each pair involved in the translocation, after the translocation is completed.)

When the meiotic process creates the gametes, these are the possible outcomes:

1. The gamete gets two normal chromosomes – no problem.
2. The gamete gets both abnormal chromosomes that traded material – no problem.
3. The gamete gets one normal and one abnormal chromosome – This will usually produce either miscarriage or a live birth with abnormalities.

Why would the third arrangement listed cause problems? Because some of the usual genetic material is missing from one of the abnormal chromosomes (due to the "lost" chunk that participated in the exchange), and some other genetic material may be duplicated (due to the material acquired from the other chromosome in the exchange that wouldn't normally be there). Whether material is missing or duplicated depends on the total number and arrangement of chromosomes contributed to the baby by each parent.

How about Robertsonian translocations? There must be problem with having only 45 autosomes, right?

Normally, there would be. In the particular case of a Robertsonian translocation, though, it is usually fine. (Remember, the only genetic material lost was the very small bits in the Mickey Mouse ears at the very end of each chromosome.)

When it comes to offspring, though, Robertsonian translocation carriers have the same problems with frequent miscarriage and sometimes abnormal offspring as the reciprocal translocation folks do – for the same reasons.

Robertsonian translocation is famous for occasionally causing what well-known syndrome?

Down syndrome (only about 4 % of the cases result from translocation, though).

Bacteria and mitochondria have their genetic material in rings. That can't happen in people, can it?

Actually, it can. If both ends of a chromosome lose a little of their material, it leaves them "sticky" or likely to bind to other similar genetic material. Sometimes, the sticky ends pick up material from other chromosomes, but occasionally, they will actually stick to each other – forming a ring.

Is having a ring chromosome a bad thing?

It depends. If only a little genetic material is lost, the phenotype will be normal or near normal. If significant genetic material is lost, the person will have a deletion or a microdeletion syndrome.

In some cases, ring chromosomes create the same picture as a partial monosomy or trisomy. A partial monosomy or trisomy situation develops as a result of cellular mechanisms that try to keep the amount of genetic material normal.

Monosomy/partial monosomy – In its effort to keep the amount of genetic material normal, the cell will sometimes break down the material it thinks is "extra" genetic material. When a ring chromosome is present, that can lead to elimination of a needed chromosome.

Trisomy/partial trisomy – Also in the effort to keep the amount of genetic material normal, cells will sometimes allow a ring chromosome to persist in a gamete, along with a normal homologous chromosome pair. Upon fertilization, the zygote then has a partial or a complete trisomy.

What is a "fragile site" on a chromosome?

An area that is especially likely to break or develop an area of allelic expansion (too many repeats of trinucleotide groupings), if the right conditions occur.

Does "Fragile X" syndrome involve a "fragile site?"

Yes – there are actually at least three fragile sites on the X chromosome associated with mental retardation. FRAXA is the fragile X syndrome site. (The others are FRAXE and FRAXF.)

What are trinucleotide repeat disorders?

"Trinucleotide repeat disorders" are disorders that develop when a particular sequence of DNA nucleotides is repeated too many times on a chromosome. For example, in fragile X syndrome, CGG triplets go from the usual number of less than 45 triplets in that location to more than 200 triplets. Depending on individual factors, when the number of triplet repeats reaches a certain threshold, the syndrome appears.

When the number of trinucleotide repeats increases, it is called "allelic expansion."

Generally, the greater the number of trinucleotide repeats, the more severe the disease or the earlier the syndrome will present.

What are some famous disorders that develop from allelic expansion of trinucleotide repeats?

Huntington's chorea, Fragile X syndrome, and myotonic dystrophy (among others)

What does "mosaicism" refer to?

When there are two or more chromosomally different cell lines in the same person, that person is genetically "mosaic." For example, some patients with a usually lethal trisomy will survive because only a portion of their cell lines have the trisomy.

How is "germ line mosaicism" different from regular (aka somatic) mosaicism?

It means that during development of the gamete cells, some lines developed an abnormal chromosomal structure. The individual who has the abnormal gametes is phenotypically normal, because the rest of his or her body cells are normal. A proportion of the gametes, though, are chromosomally abnormal, putting the individual at risk for multiple affected offspring or miscarriages.

If mosaicism is suspected, what study is required to confirm it?

The chromosomal structure of fibroblasts must be checked – lymphocytes may also be checked, *but they may give a false negative.*

> A false-negative result from lymphocyte studies can occur for two reasons. First, the lymphocyte is derived from a different cell line than the fibroblast. One cell population might have the abnormal form, while the other does not. Second, lymphocytes are more likely to "correct" genetic errors than fibroblasts are. Mosaicism might have actually affected both cell types, but the lymphocytes "edited" their genome to fix it, while the fibroblasts did not.

> Example – Hypomelanosis of Ito is a particularly nice example of a mosaic disorder. In this disorder, the mosaic cell lines affect certain patches of skin, but not others. The mosaicism in the skin is visually clear, because the skin has different levels of pigment in the abnormal skin, so the color of affected skin and normal skin is different. Sometimes, there are associated abnormalities of the eyes, central nervous system, and musculoskeletal system.

Uniparental disomy and uniparental isodisomy: Help! What are these?

Uniparental disomy means that someone with a normal number of chromosomes inherited both chromosomes of one chromosome pair *from the same parent*. This is not supposed to happen!

This shouldn't be possible. How could it happen?

There are two ways –

Uniparental isodisomy means that both copies of the abnormally inherited pair are identical. The isodisomy phenomenon usually occurs when a gamete inherits only one chromosome of a pair, and, in an effort to fix the situation, the single chromosome is copied.

Uniparental heterodisomy means that both homologues of the chromosome pair were inherited from the same parent, but they were the two different chromosomes carried by that parent.

Example – The most famous examples of uniparental disomy are Angelman syndrome and Prader–Willi syndrome. (*Please remember, though, that this is not the only way these syndromes can develop. They also result from deletions on chromosome 15, combined with imprinting – see below.*)

Prader–Willi develops when chromosome 15 is inherited as a uniparental disomy from the mother, and Angelman syndrome develops when the uniparental disomy comes from the father. These syndromes can result from either isodisomy or heterodisomy.

You explained how uniparental isodisomy can happen. What about uniparental heterodisomy?

Usually, it occurs because trisomy was present at some point in development. The embryo, in any effort to save itself (called trisomy rescue), eliminated some of the abnormal genetic material but unfortunately kept two copies from the same parent.

What is imprinting?

When a disorder has genomic imprinting as part of its inheritance pattern, it means that the disorder you observe depends on whether the mother or the father contributed the faulty gene sequence.

Prader–Willi and Angelman syndromes occur due to both uniparental disomy and deletions on chromosome 15. When the cause is a deletion on chromosome 15, then the imprinting phenomenon is observed – Prader–Willi develops when the paternal chromosome 15 has the deletion (just as it develops when there is uniparental disomy of the mother's chromosome 15 – missing the father's input in chromosome 15 causes Prader–Willi). If the maternal chromosome 15 has a deletion, Angelman syndrome is the result.

Mnemonic for what's missing in Prader–Willi:

Prader sounds like pater, vader, fader – all words that can mean father in various languages. Developing Prader–Willi means that the "father" is missing. The Catholic church is having a difficult time recruiting priests these days – think of a church without a "father" to remember that Prader–Willi comes from missing paternal genes.

Other techniques to study chromosomal disorders include the following:

– FISH: Fluorescent in situ hybridization uses fluorescent probes to bind to regions of interest on the chromosome. This can be used to diagnose microdeletions or duplications, such as in DiGeorge syndrome.
– Chromosomal microarray (CMA, array CGH) is a technique to look at genomic copy number variations in more detail than a karyotype can provide. DNA from the patient's sample and a normal reference sample are labeled differently, using different fluorescent colors, and hybridized to several thousand probes. The genetic probes used include most of the known genes and noncoding regions of the genome, printed on a glass slide. The fluorescent intensity of the patient's DNA vs. the reference DNA is compared. The copy number changes for a particular location in the genome can then be estimated by measuring the difference in intensities in the two samples. ***CMA is recommended as the first-line test in the investigation of a child with intellectual disability and/or multiple congenital anomalies.***

(FISH, an older technique, tests for one region per probe, whereas CMA tests for the entire genome at once.)

Genetic Gems

If an inherited disorder is being transmitted through the *mitochondria*, the mother is always affected, and *all* of the children must be affected. After all, they can only get their mitochondria from their Mom.

(In real life, mitochondrial disorders are a little more complicated, and some do arise from new mutations.)

Dominant (aka autosomal dominant) disorders are **bold**! Just one copy of the bad gene is enough for it to show itself – it's not shy, so it doesn't need company. About 50 % of offspring are affected by autosomal dominant disorders, and both girls and boys are equally affected.

Recessive disorders (aka autosomal recessive) are shy! They won't show themselves unless there are two recessive genes present. These disorders often "skip" generations, because only one bad gene was present in the various family members, so no one knew they had a bad gene.

If a disorder is "*X-linked*," that just means that the abnormal gene is on the X chromosome – the problem gene can still be either dominant or recessive. What we typically think of as X-linked disorders are really X-linked recessive disorders.

X-linked recessive disorders generally occur in males (because they have only one X chromosome, so the bad gene's effect is unopposed). Affected males will never pass the disorder to their sons, because their sons only received the Y chromosome from Dad. (Rarely, a female can be affected if she happens to inherit two bad copies of the gene – one on each of her X chromosomes, just as could happen with any recessive disorder – or if the female has Turner syndrome and therefore has only one X chromosome.)

Oddly enough, an *X-linked dominant* disorder will occur more often in females, because they have more X chromosomes. Their likelihood of getting one bad X chromosome is therefore higher. Daughters of a man who has an X-linked dominant disorder will *always* be affected, because he has only one X chromosome to give to all of his daughters.

(X-linked dominant disorders are not common. The classic example is a disorder called incontinentia pigmenti, characterized by hyperpigmented whorls on the skin and abnormalities of the eyes and teeth.)

What is X inactivation? (Discovered by Mary Lyon, hence the term "lyonization")

Humans are only meant to have a certain amount of genetic material. If we have too much or too little, a disorder usually occurs. This presents a problem because men and women have a different amount of genetic material due to the X chromosome being bigger than the Y chromosome.

The species deals with this by partially inactivating one of the Xs in the females. Early in development, the various cells choose which X will be inactivated – it is not the same for all of the cells. The partially inactivated X chromosome shrinks up, forming the small, dense, object known as the "Barr body." The loci (gene locations) that are present on the Y chromosome are still active on the Barr body. The extra genes, though, are inactive.

All of the daughter cells that result from division of the early cells will have the same inactivated X as their mother cell. This means that women are always a genetic mosaic, with some cells having one X chromosome fully active, while other cells having the opposite X fully active.

Chapter 2
Selected Genetics Topics

Robertsonian Translocation and Other Travel Options for Your Genes: How Your Genes Can do a Little Sightseeing on the Genome

Some chromosome problems have to do with the number of chromosomes – either too many, or not enough, compared to the usual 23 pairs. Other chromosome problems have to do with loss or gain of genetic material, compared to usual (such as deletion disorders), without any change in the usual organization of the chromosome.

A final category of chromosomal disorders is related to the chromosomal *structure* or placement of the genes, rather than the total number of chromosomes or the total amount of genetic material.

Robertsonian translocations fall into this "structural" category.

How Do Chromosomes Mess up their Structure?

Chromosome structure problems occur when chromosomes break and then reattach. If they rejoin at the same place they left, the process is called "*restitution*." If they rejoin the chromosome in a new location, the process is called "*reunion*."

Generally, pieces of broken chromosome attach to places in the chromosomes where a break has occurred. The ends of broken chromosomes are "sticky," so they tend to attach to each other, whether the other sticky end is their original site or not.

When a *reunion* occurs (new site of attachment), the new arrangement may be "**balanced**," meaning that the same amount of genetic material normally present in human cells will still be present and no clinical problems are likely to occur for that individual.

C.M. Houser, *Pediatric Genetics and Inborn Errors of Metabolism:*
A Practically Painless Review, DOI 10.1007/978-1-4939-0581-2_2,
© Springer Science+Business Media New York 2014

Alternatively, the reunion could produce an "**unbalanced" translocation**. An unbalanced translocation means that genetic material was either gained or lost. When an unbalanced translocation occurs during meiosis, the individual who develops from that gamete is usually affected by some clinical problems.

Balanced translocations

There are three types of balanced translocations, meaning translocations that preserve the total amount of genetic material correctly but alter the usual structure of the chromosome.

1. Balanced reciprocal translocations
   Two nonhomologous (not the same) chromosomes exchange segments. Amount of material is the same, and the individual is usually fine. Gametes produced by an individual with a balanced reciprocal translocation are often abnormal, however. (So, for example, miscarriages are more frequent in this population.)

2. Inversions
   A section of a chromosome *flips around* so that it is facing the opposite direction in the chromosome. The individual is usually fine, and gametes are often fine, but occasionally abnormal.

3. Robertsonian translocations
   Robertsonian translocations are a special case of *unequal* reciprocal translocation.

   Two acrocentric (the centromere joins the two parts close to one end of the chromosome) chromosomes form a new metacentric (joined in the middle) chromosome. They fuse near their original centromere location and lose the very short arms in the process. These short portions of the chromosome are usually nonfunctional, so the loss doesn't cause problems for the individual who has it. As usual, the offspring are at increased risk for problems.

   The new translocation chromosome is made up of the long arms of two fused chromosomes – which means that the individual now has only 45 chromosomes!

Ring chromosomes

Deletion at each end of a chromosome allows the two ends to fuse into a ring! This can happen because the exposed rings are sticky, and sometimes they form a reunion *with each other*.

People born with ring chromosomes can be normal, near normal, or may have a variety of congenital anomalies and/or mental retardation.

For people who are affected by a ring chromosome, their phenotype is similar to individuals with a similar monosomy – depending on the quantity of genetic material lost.

Trisomy 21: Just the Facts, Please!

The majority of Trisomy 21 births are to mothers in what age group?

The 20s – they have more babies than older age groups and are less likely to be screened for trisomies.

What prenatal screening pattern suggests a Trisomy 21 fetus?

↓ AFP
↓ Estriol
↓ HCG

What ultrasound findings suggest Trisomy 21?

Thickened nuchal (neck) skin fold
Short or missing nasal bone
Short femur
+ Cardiac and GI abnormalities, of course (e.g., endocardial cushion defects, duodenal atresia)

Much has been made of translocation as a cause for Down syndrome. What's up with that?

Folks in medicine always get excited when we figure something out, so there is now a lot of talk about translocation as a cause for Down syndrome. It is true that translocation can cause Down syndrome, but the vast majority of Down syndrome patients have trisomy, *not translocation.*

The breakdown of Down syndrome causes is:

95 %:   Three copies of chromosome 21 (trisomy)
 1 %:   Mosaic
 4 %:   Translocations

Translocation as a cause of Down syndrome is more common in younger mothers (less than 30 years old).

Half of the translocations are inherited – half are new translocations specific to that gamete.

Not all of the translocations that produce Down syndrome involve chromosome 21 alone. Sometimes other chromosomes, such as number 14, are part of the translocation process.

Parents of Down syndrome infants due to translocation should have chromosomal evaluation. Why?

To find out whether they have a translocation or not. The risk of Down recurring in a future pregnancy cannot be calculated unless you first know whether one of the parents has a translocation and which one.

The worst possible translocation to have is a 21q21q translocation. These parents have only two possibilities in offspring – autosomal monosomy (no chromosome 21q arms, which results in a nonviable fetus) or Down syndrome infants due to three copies of the q arm of chromosome 21 (two from the translocation parent and one from the presumably normal parent).

Risk of recurrence due to a parental translocation can vary depending on whether the Mom or the Dad has the translocation (oddly enough).

Chapter 3
General Genetics Question and Answer Items

Is advanced paternal age associated with genetic disorders?	**Yes –** **paternal age of ≥ 35 years**
What sort of genetic disorders are mainly associated with advanced *maternal* age?	**Chromosomal disorders**
What sort of genetic disorders are mainly associated with advanced *paternal* age?	New mutations
If a couple has a child with a genetic disorder, and advanced paternal age was a likely factor, what can you tell the couple about the probability of recurrence in future siblings?	We can't predict it, currently
What is the hallmark of X-linked inheritance on the family pedigree?	**No male-to-male transmission**
What is the classic example of an X-linked dominant disorder?	Incontinentia pigmenti (whorls of pigment, often with dental & oculomotor abnormalities)
What will you see if a disorder is inherited as an X-linked dominant disorder?	Both girls and boys are affected (and a higher percentage is affected than in a recessive disorder – roughly 50 %)

C.M. Houser, *Pediatric Genetics and Inborn Errors of Metabolism:*
A Practically Painless Review, DOI 10.1007/978-1-4939-0581-2_3,
© Springer Science+Business Media New York 2014

What is "germ line" mosaicism?	**When a proportion of the germ cells (sperm or eggs) are different chromosomally from the others**
What is (plain old) mosaicism?	**When a single individual has two or more chromosomal compositions (in different cell lines)**
How does mosaicism usually happen?	A trisomy or other chromosomal problem happens, but some of the cells correct it (They will "eat" extra chromosomal material, or create missing chromosomal material, in some cases)
What is uniparental isodisomy?	**When both copies of a chromosome come from one parent and the copies are identical** **(Usually occurs when one chromosome was missing and the zygote corrected that by copying the chromosome it had)**
What is uniparental heterodisomy?	**When both copies of a chromosome come from one parent and the copies are different** **(Both of the chromosomes the parent had were transmitted, so they are not identical)**
Most Down syndrome children are the result of chromosomal nondisjunction. If there is a 21/21 translocation, though, what is the risk of recurrence?	**100 %**
What is the risk of a couple having another child with Down syndrome, if one parent has a 14/21 translocation?	Depends on which parent has it – Mom = 14 % Dad = 4 %
What percentage of Down syndrome cases is due to trisomy 21?	**95 %**

What are the two major teratogenic effects of ACE inhibitors?

Skull and kidney defects

What teratogenic effect is sometimes observed with hyperthermia (e.g., sitting in the hot tub while pregnant)?

Neural tube defects

How common is fetal alcohol syndrome in the USA?

1 per 500 births!

What is the typical facial appearance in fetal alcohol syndrome (FAS)?

- **Flat philtrum**
- **Thin upper lip**
- **Mid-face hypoplasia with a short & broad nose**

(the philtrum is the area between the upper lip and nose)

If a Mom has one infant affected by FAS, what is the usual pattern for future offspring?

If Mom continues to drink, the phenotype worsens with each successive child

(liver may be processing the alcohol less easily as time goes by, so effects increase)

What is the genetic phenomenon of "imprinting?"

When a different result is expected from the same genetic error, depending on whether the genetic error comes from the Mom or the Dad

One example of imprinting is the hydatidiform mole. How is this an example of imprinting?

Triploidy from the father can result in hydatidiform mole

(Triploidy from the mother would not)

Most of the trinucleotide repeats that cause well-known disorders have which nucleotides in the first and third positions?

C and G
(position 1 and position 3, respectively)

Which trinucleotide repeat produces fragile X syndrome?

CGG
(think of the "g" in fraGile, to remember it's in the middle position)

Even though fragile X syndrome results from a trinucleotide repeat, what inheritance pattern does it follow?	X-linked recessive
What are the hallmarks of fragile X on physical exam? (3)	1. Big ears 2. Big testes (after puberty) 3. MR
Which trinucleotide repeat produces myotonic dystrophy?	CTG (think of the "t" in myoTonic dysTrophy)
Which trinucleotide repeat produces Huntington's disease?	CAG (think of the bAsAl gAngliA to remember that "A" is important)
Plexiform neurofibromas in neurofibromatosis can develop into what sort of malignancy?	**Neurofibrosarcomas**
Female neurofibromatosis patients tend to have significant worsening of their disease in what situations?	Pregnancy & puberty
Why are plexiform neurofibromas problematic?	**They sometimes hypertrophy, become malignant, and compress other structures**
There are three types of neurofibromas, plexiform, nodular, and cutaneous. What is the main trouble with the nodular form?	Compression of nerves
Cutaneous fibromas sometimes cause what symptomatic problems for patients?	**Itching or pain**
What symptoms are most common for NF-2 patients?	**Hearing loss Other sensory problems Unsteadiness (not many neurofibromas)**
What kind of routine evaluation will Marfan's patients need?	**Echocardiography (to monitor the aortic root – risk of aortic dilatation and dissection)**

Which gene is abnormal in Marfan's syndrome?

Fibrillin (FBN1)

(Transforming growth factor – beta receptor 2 has also been identified. TOO NEW for boards)

What is the classic description of the scarring that sometimes occurs for patients with Ehlers–Danlos syndrome?

Cigarette paper scarring

Pierre–Robin sequence, combined with deafness, eye problems, and Marfanoid habitus, means you are probably dealing with what genetic disorder?

Stickler syndrome (autosomal dominant connective tissue disorder)

Stickler syndrome is a heterogeneous genetic disorder. What does that mean?

Several different genes/chromosomes cause the same syndrome

What proportion of Pierre–Robin patients actually have Stickler syndrome?

1/3

What is the typical facial appearance of Stickler syndrome, and what is the main system the syndrome affects?

- Flat face/mid-face hypoplasia
- Special senses (eyes & hearing)

If Stickler patients have a Marfanoid habitus, do they have joint problems, too?

Yes – hypermobility and arthropathy

Retinitis pigmentosa + sensorineural hearing loss = what syndrome?

Usher syndrome

Mnemonic:
Think of an usher in a movie theatre who is both blind & deaf!

The hands of achondroplastic patients are often described as "trident hands." What does that mean?

Fingers are short, with a broad base that tapers out to a narrow fingertip

(The broad base makes the fingers stick out away from each other, so it looks a bit like a trident)

When we're talking about disorders with shorts limbs, what term indicates that the *proximal* part of the limb is the short part?	**Rhizomelic (for example, achondroplasia)**
If a disorder has shortened limbs, and the middle segment of the limb is the short part, what is that called?	Mesomelic
Although it doesn't come up as often as the other types of limb shortening, what is the term for a shortened distal segment of the limb?	Acromelic
Beaked nose, with prominent forehead and eyes, suggests what genetic disorder?	**Crouzon syndrome** (They look like they're cruisin' at high speed in a cartoon – the forehead & eyes are forward, while the lower face recedes a bit)
Facial angiofibromas are a problem in tuberous sclerosis. What is their usual distribution on the face?	**Butterfly distribution, although the individual lesions look similar to acne (absolute favorite spot is alar crease)**
Which cardiac tumor suggests the tuberous sclerosis diagnosis?	**Cardiac rhabdomyomas**
Are tuberous sclerosis carriers symptomatic?	Often not symptomatic
What are the usual head CT findings for tuberous sclerosis patients?	• **Intracerebral "tubers"** – **the buzzword for their appearance is "candle drippings"** • **Periventricular calcified tubers**
Tuberous sclerosis patients are often recognized by their skin findings. What ophthalmological findings do they usually also have?	• Spots on the optic nerve called "mulberry tumors" • Flat, gray spots on the disk called "phakomas"

Is it common for Sturge–Weber patients to have mental retardation?	**Yes**
A patient is presented with seizures, hemiparesis, MR, and intracerebral calcifications. What is the likely diagnosis?	**Sturge–Weber** (the calcifications follow the gyral pattern of the brain, underneath the area with the port-wine stain)
What is a "genotype?"	**Description of the particular genes an individual has**
What is the "phenotype?"	**The consequences of a particular genetic makeup in a particular individual**
For a disorder to be considered hereditary, what is required?	The disorder can be passed in the genes from parent to child
How is a familial disorder different from a hereditary disorder?	**Anything that "clusters" in a family can be called "familial" (including infectious disease!)**
What is the "penetrance" of a genetic disorder?	**The percent of cases in which individuals who have the genes for the disease actually develop the disease**
How is "expression" of the gene different from "penetrance?"	**"Penetrance" is all or none – either the individual develops the disease or not** **"Expression" is the specific way the disorder shows itself in different individuals**
What is the typical boards example of a disorder with variable penetrance?	**Retinoblastoma (10 % of those with the gene don't develop the disorder)**
What is the penetrance of retinoblastoma?	90 % (10 % don't develop it)
What is pleiotropy?	**A single gene creating problems for more than one system (having more than one effect)**

How is pleiotropy different from variable expression?	Pleiotropy means the gene affects more than one system – Variable expression means that the way it affects the system can be different in different individuals
How is Treacher–Collins syndrome an example of variable expression?	Some children have cleft palate, and some do not
The particular forms a gene can take are called _____?	Alleles
How many alleles do humans have, for each gene location?	Two
If both genes coding for a particular trait are the same, that individual is _____ for the trait (e.g., blue eye color)?	Homozygous
Two different alleles at a particular locus is called _____?	Heterozygous
If a pedigree drawing shows that a disorder can be passed from father to son, what does that tell you about inheritance?	1. It is *not* X-linked 2. It is not mitochondrial
If a disorder is autosomal dominant, then every affected child will have what in the pedigree?	An affected parent (Unless there is a new mutation, of course – but boards exams usually don't show pedigrees of a new mutation)
If a disorder is autosomal recessive, and two carriers (heterozygotes) mate, what is the probability of producing affected offspring?	25 %
If a father has an X-linked recessive disorder, what is his probability of passing the disease gene to his daughters?	100 % (He has only one X, which is affected, and daughters get one of their Xs from their fathers)

Can an X-linked recessive disorder be transmitted from father to son?

No –
A male child cannot get an X chromosome from his Dad, only the Y

If a mother carries a defective X chromosome (in a carrier state), what is the probability that she will pass it on to her child?

50 %

(Either X could end up in the new embryo – whether it's male or female)

If a disorder is transmitted as an X-linked <u>dominant</u> disorder (very unusual), what proportion of the children will be affected?

50 % – both boys and girls will be affected because the disorder is dominant

Can an x-linked recessive disorder "skip" a generation?

Yes –
If only females are born

(or if the males born just happen to get lucky, but there are still some female carriers born)

Which female genetic disorder would result in females being symptomatic for X-linked recessive disorders?

Turner's – They only have one X!

In what sense are females always "somatic mosaics?"

One X is randomly chosen for inactivation in each female cell. There are therefore two populations of somatic cells in females

In some cases, female carriers of X-linked recessive disorders show at least partial manifestations of the disorder. Why is that?

Somatic mosaicism –
Some of the female's cells are using only the "bad copy" of the X chromosome

In general, it doesn't matter which parent supplies a particular gene to a child. Are there ever situations in which it does?

Yes – genomic imprinting

Give a classic example of genomic imprinting.

Prader–Willi & Angelman syndrome –

Deletion of the same gene portion causes Prader–Willi if it comes from the father but Angelman syndrome if it comes from the Mom!

Can both copies of a chromosome come from the same parent?	**Yes –** **It's called uniparental disomy**
How does uniparental disomy happen?	**Chromosomes fail to separate (nondisjunction) → one trisomic & one monosomic cell** **The cells try to fix themselves, by copying or destroying a chromosome, and end up with two copies of the same chromosome**
Mitochondrial diseases are inherited from which parent?	**Mother <u>only</u>**
What does homoplasmy and heteroplasmy refer to in the mitochondrial population?	Whether all mitochondria in the cell have the same DNA or not
How does heteroplasmy occur for mitochondrial DNA?	The mitochondria replicate independently – If a DNA error is made in one, the others are still normal, but now there are two (DNA) groups
If a genetic disease is due to "multifactorial inheritance," what does that mean?	**Multiple genes affect the likelihood of a particular disorder happening**
In multifactorial disorders, what are "liability" factors?	**Bad genes that contribute to the likelihood of developing the disorder**
What is a "liability threshold" in multifactorial genetic disease?	**The number of liability factors that must be present for a disease to become manifest**
In some cases, the liability threshold for a multifactorial disorder can be different for males vs. females. What is a classic example of this phenomenon?	**Pyloric stenosis –** **Females require many more liability factors to develop the disease than males do**

Who is more likely to "pass on" pyloric stenosis to his or her offspring – a mother who had it or a father?

Mother –
She had to have many liability factors to develop it, but male children need only a few liability factors to get it!

If a child is born to a parent who had pyloric stenosis, which gender of child is most likely to have pyloric stenosis?

Males
(They only need a few liability factors to develop the disorder)

In multifactorial diseases, what is the relationship between the severity of a disease in an affected family member and the likelihood of other family members being affected?

Worse severity = greater likelihood other family members will be affected

Increasing numbers of affected family members _____ the probability of subsequent affected family members being born in multifactorial genetic diseases.

Increases

The main factors that determine how likely family members are to be affected by a multifactorial genetic disease are _____?
(5)

1. # of family members affected
2. Less commonly affected gender has been affected (↑ risk)
3. Severity in affected individual(s)
4. Degree of relationship (closeness of the kindred)
5. Prevalence in the general population

Dizygotic twins share what percentage of their genetic material?

About 50 %
(same as any other siblings)

Monozygotic twins share what percentage of their genetic material?

100 %

If a particular disorder is more commonly shared by monozygotic twins than it is by dizygotic twins, this strongly suggests that the disorder is at least partly due to _____?

Genetics

The main clue that a couple is at risk for producing children with a genetic disorder is _____?

Family history of genetic disorder

Translocation has gotten a lot of attention as a way that Down syndrome can occur. What percentage of Down syndrome cases are due to translocation?	**About 3 %** (precise number varies in different sources)
What percentage of Down syndrome cases are due to a whole, extra, chromosome 21?	**94 %**
So, some Down syndrome cases are due to trisomy 21, and some are due to translocation, but when you add up the numbers you don't get 100 %. What accounts for the remaining Down syndrome cases?	**3 % due to mosaicism** (precise number varies in different sources) (94 % trisomy) (3 % translocation)
What is the only known risk factor for trisomy 21?	**Advanced maternal age**
How does trisomy 21 occur?	**Nondisjunction during meiosis**
What should you advise as appropriate Down syndrome screening for women <35 years old?	**The "triple" screen** ↓ **AFP** ↓ **Unconjugated estriol** ↑ **HCG** (In current practice, you may see more factors being added)
What is brachydactyly (often seen in Down syndrome)?	Short, broad, fingers
Some other common & obvious findings of Down syndrome are _____? (Five main ones – there are certainly others)	1. **Small ears & head** 2. **Mental retardation** 3. **Hypotonia** 4. **Simian crease on palm** 5. **Epicanthal fold**
Which other significant problems are very common in Down syndrome? (5) (1 malignancy) (1 mechanical problem) (3 organ problems)	1. **GI (duodenal atresia & Hirschsprung's, in particular)** 2. **Heart (A-V canal or VSD problems)** 3. **Leukemia** 4. **Atlanto-axial instability** 5. **Hypothyroidism**

What proportion of Down syndrome kids have congenital heart defects?	**50 %**
What types of cardiac problems do Down syndrome kids most often have?	VSD (1/3) A-V canal issues (1/3) Tetralogy of Fallot & ASDs (1/3)
What is the buzzword for the types of ASD & VSD problems often seen in Down syndrome?	**"Endocardial cushion defect"**
If Down syndrome patients have GI anomalies, they usually present clinically. What X-ray finding should you look for in Down syndrome babies with feeding issues?	**Double-bubble** (for duodenal atresia – one stomach bubble and one duodenal bubble)
What especially photogenic facial finding is sometimes a photo item for Down syndrome?	**Brushfield spots –** **Speckled spots on the iris**
Which type of leukemia is most common in Down patients?	**ALL**
Why might a Down syndrome baby have an abnormal white blood cell count early in infancy – while healthy?	**"Transient" abnormal myelopoiesis** (spontaneously resolves, usually by 3 months old)
When should you check for atlanto-axial instability in a Down syndrome patient?	About age 3 (before preschool)
What is the recommended protocol for screening Down syndrome patients for hypothyroidism?	Screen at birth, 6, & 12 months – then annually
What special screening studies should you do for your Down syndrome patients? **(4)**	1. **Cardiac echo (ASAP)** 2. **Thyroid studies** 3. **Ophtho screen <6 months** 4. **Hearing screen <6 months**
Abnormalities of the sex chromosomes are the most common chromosomal abnormality. Among autosomal (non-sex) chromosomes, what is the most common abnormality?	Trisomy 21

If a mother has a Down syndrome (trisomy 21) baby, how likely is she to have another?

1 % if she is <35 years old

For mothers >35 years old, how likely are they to have a second Down's child, if they already have one Down's child?

It varies with age – they have approximately double the risk as other Moms their age

If a couple has a Down syndrome infant due to a translocation, what are the chances of the next infant also having Down's?

Depends on the translocation

Is trisomy 18 more common in boys or girls?

Girls!
(4:1)

What do children with trisomy 18 usually die of?

Central apnea

All trisomies occur more often with increasing _____?

**Maternal age
(mainly >35 years)**

If a Mom <35 years old has a child with a trisomy, the risk of her next child having that same trisomy is _____?

1 %

How long do Edwards syndrome (trisomy 18) children usually live?

<1 year

**The most characteristic findings for Edwards syndrome (trisomy 18) are _____?
(2)**

**Rocker bottom feet/club foot
Clenched fist**
(kind of the same thing)

There are two ways that Patau's syndrome can occur. What are they?

1. Trisomy 13
2. Unbalanced translocation → three copies of 13q

**What characteristics do you expect to find on exam of a trisomy 13 patient?
(Five main ones)**

1. **Orofacial cleft/cleft lip**
2. **Holoprosencephaly
   (mid-face/CNS defects)**
3. **Microphthalmia**
4. **Genital abnormalities**
5. **Hypoplastic or absent ribs**

Children who survive (long term) with trisomy 13 usually <u>don't</u> have which feature?	Holoprosencephaly
What thoracic finding is common in trisomy 13 (Patau's)?	**Absent or hypoplastic ribs**
How common are cardiac problems with Patau's syndrome, trisomy 13?	Very common – 80 % have them
Infants with trisomy 8 are usually not viable. Those that are usually have what type of trisomy 8?	Mosaic (not all cells affected)
Characteristic facial features with trisomy 8 are _____ & _____?	• High forehead • Thick & everted lower lip
Trisomy 8 children are at increased risk for what malignancy?	AML
The long arm of a chromosome is designated with what letter?	**q**
What letter designates the short arm of a chromosome?	**p**
"Deletion" genetic syndromes usually present with some typical physical phenotype findings, and what else?	**Mental retardation**
"4p-" deletion causes what syndrome?	Wolf–Hirschhorn (Think of a wolf going <u>4</u> a "<u>Pee</u>" in the woods!)
Wolf–Hirschhorn syndrome usually has what developmental consequences?	<u>Severe</u> **developmental delay**

What is the most noted physical finding in Wolf–Hirschhorn syndrome (4p-)?

"Greek helmet" facies (Glabella is prominent & eyes are set wide apart. Picasso also liked to do profiles this way!)

It is very common for Wolf–Hirschhorn patients to have what neurological problem?

Seizures
(90 %)

Fifty-percent of Wolf–Hirschhorn patients have abnormalities of what important organ?

The heart

What are the buzzwords for the facial appearance of Wolf–Hirschhorn patients?

"Greek helmet" facies
Prominent glabella
Frontal bossing
Ocular hypertelorism
   (means wide-set eyes)

Aside from a characteristic facial appearance, what else goes with Wolf–Hirschhorn?
(3)

Seizures
Severe developmental delay
Heart anomalies

A wolf peeing in the woods is supposed to make you think of _____?

The genetic defect causing Wolf–Hirschhorn – (4p-)

What is unusual about the cry of a child with 5p- deletion?

Sounds like a cat
(due to anatomic changes in the larynx)

What is the other name for 5p- deletion?

Cri-du-chat
(Cry of the cat, for the non-French speakers in the group)

What are the main facial characteristics of Cri-du-chat patients?

1. "Moon face" with wide-set eyes
2. Downward slanted palpebral fissures
3. Wide, flat nasal bridge

Mnemonic:
Think of a Persian <u>cat</u> – they have a round face, flat nasal bridge, and downgoing palpebral fissures. Just make the nose & eyes a little wide!

In addition to the facial features of Cri-du-chat, what other findings are typical for the head?
(2)

1. Microcephaly
2. High, arched palate

What sort of cognitive function is typical for Cri-du-chat patients?

MR
(mental retardation – Some say Persian cats aren't too smart!)

What is abnormal about the muscles of Cri-du-chat patients?

Hypotonic
(Persian cats don't exercise much, so their muscles are hypotonic)

Are Cri-du-chat patients typically tall or short?

Short

A short, floppy baby, with a round face and small head – featuring a flat nasal bridge & widely spaced eyes – is likely to have what genetic disorder?

5p-/Cri-du-chat

Are cardiac problems frequent in Cri-du-chat patients?

Yes –
1/3 of patients have them

How can you remember the underlying genetic issue in Cri-du-chat syndrome?

If cats are supposed to have nine lives, then these kids have used up <u>5</u> of them just making it to the delivery room! (5p-)

A child with *atretic or narrowed ear canals* is a classic presentation of which genetic syndrome?

De Grouchy (18q-)

Mnemonic:
Because not hearing well can make you grouchy!

Which genetic boo-boo causes de Grouchy syndrome?

18q- (deletion)

Mnemonic:
Think of a grouchy 18-year-old – he's grouchy because he is "minus" his voter registration. He couldn't hear the announcement to get in the "queue" due to narrow ear canals!

What is unusual about the mouth of de Grouchy syndrome (18q-) patients?

It looks like a goldfish mouth (carp mouth – everted lower lip)

(Note: Other genetic disorders also have this finding, such as trisomy 8)

Do de Grouchy syndrome patients have normal intellect?

No –
mentally retarded

(Remember that most deletions produce some level of MR)

Describe the face of a de Grouchy syndrome patient.

**Mid-face pushed in
Mandible protrudes
Goldfish mouth
Deep-set eyes**

What is unusual about the legs of de Grouchy (18q-) infants?

They are usually held in a frog-legged position

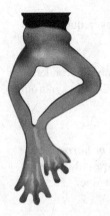

A child is presented with a protruding mouth and jaw, but receding eyes & mid-face. The external auditory meatus is not patent. What is the disorder?

De Grouchy (18q-)

Trigonocephaly (triangle head) goes with what genetic problem?

9p-

What other physical finding is very prominent in 9p- patients?

Pterygium colli
(A bilateral tight band of tissue running from the mastoid to the acromion)

Mnemonic:
Think of the pterygium as extending the triangle of the head down to the shoulders

Hypoplastic hands, that look like a mitten (often missing the thumbs, & with other fingers often syndactylous), go with what genetic disorder?

13q-

Mnemonic:
Think of a group of 13 "performing mittens" who have just missed their "cue" to go onstage!

What is unusual about the 18q- deletion disorder?

80 % are basically normal
(minor mr & minor physical anomalies)

What is a microdeletion?

Loss of a single gene or a few contiguous genes

Can microdeletions result in genetic disorders?

Sure!

Can microdeletions be detected in the usual chromosome preparations?

No –
They're too small to create a visible difference in the size of the chromosome arm

What is the best test to detect a microdeletion?

Chromosomal microarray (CMA)

What famous pair of disorders results from a single microdeletion that has different effects depending on whether it came from Mom or Dad?

Prader–Willi

&

Angelman Syndrome

What microdeletion produces both Prader–Willi and Angelman syndrome?

15q11–13

Seizures, severe MR, fair hair, and jerky ataxic movements (along with bout of laughter) indicate what microdeletion syndrome?

Angelman

(Happy puppet)

At birth, an infant has small hands & feet and hypotonia. What microdeletion syndrome should you think of?

Prader–Willi

(15q11–13)

As a Prader–Willi patient grows up, what characteristics usually develop?

Short & fat
Mild MR
Small gonads

Prader–Willi develops when the 15q11–13 microdeletion is inherited from which parent?

Dad

Mnemonic:
"Prader" sounds like "pater," the Latin word for father!

When a 15q11–13 microdeletion is inherited from the mother, what syndrome results?

Angelman

Mnemonic:
… because women are angels!

What is pseudohypogonadism, and which genetic disorder is it associated with?

- Gonads are normal sized, but the body is abnormally large

- Laurence–Moon–Biedl syndrome

What are the two main clues that a patient may have Laurence–Moon–Biedl syndrome?

- Pseudohypogonadism

- Significant gynecomastia

(So the patient seems big, but feminized, until you get out the orchidometer!)

What named gene is missing in Williams syndrome?

Elastin – chromosome 7
(one copy is missing)

What type of disorder is Williams syndrome?

Microdeletion of 7q11.23-

What are the main features of Williams syndrome?

- **Friendly, "cocktail party" personality**
- **Aortic stenosis (supravalvular)**

Do Williams syndrome patients have normal cognition?

No –
They have MR

The facial findings of Williams syndrome mainly have to do with what part of the face?

Eyes

What are the facial findings of Williams syndrome?

Stellate iris pattern
(*starlike*)
Strabismus
Periorbital fullness

What are the features of WAGR syndrome?

Wilms tumor
Aniridia
Genital hypoplasia
Retardation (mental)

11p13- is a microdeletion syndrome. What is the name of the syndrome?

WAGR syndrome

Microdeletion of which two genes causes WAGR syndrome (if either is missing)?

PAX 6
  or
Wilms
tumor 1
gene

Both PAX 6 & Wilms tumor 1 genes are found on which chromosome?

11 (short arm)

Which GI syndrome, involving a paucity of bile ducts, can be a microdeletion disorder?

Alagille syndrome

(Most Alagille patients have a point mutation)

What are the main features expected in Alagille syndrome?

1. **Bile duct paucity**
2. **Pulmonary valve & pulmonary artery stenosis**
3. **Triangular faces**
4. **Butterfly vertebrae**

What gene, specifically, causes Alagille syndrome if it mutates?

Jagged-1
(Chromosome 20)

Mnemonic:
Think of jagged butterfly vertebrae damaging the bile ducts

What are the most common cardiac system abnormalities in Alagille syndrome?

Pulmonary stenosis

&

Tetralogy of Fallot

What ocular abnormality is often seen in Alagille syndrome but rarely causes symptoms?

Posterior "embryotoxon"

(a prominent eye ring
& iris stranding)

Is "posterior embryotoxon" related to a "toxin" or toxic something?

No –
It's a developmental abnormality

Which microdeletion causes Di George syndrome and a group of related disorders?

22q11.2-

What is a good mnemonic for the findings associated with the 22q11.2 deletion?

CATCH 22
Cleft palate
Absent Thymus
Congenital Heart disease

What are the main general conse-quences of 22q11.2 microdeletion?
(3)

1. **Immune deficiencies**
2. **Hypocalcemia**
3. **Cardiac anomalies**

(both 1 & 2 are thymus related)

How is cognition affected by the 22q11.2 microdeletion?

Learning disabilities are common (2/3 of patients), & some have MR

Embryologically speaking, what is the problem in 22q11.2 microdeletion?

Development of 3rd & 4th pharyngeal pouches is abnormal

What are the four most common cardiac problems in 22q11.2 microdeletion?
(in descending order)

1. **Tetralogy of Fallot**
2. **Interrupted aortic arch**
3. **VSD**
4. **Truncus arteriosus**

How do Di George syndrome patients often come to medical attention?

Seizure due to hypocalcemia

How common is it to have the wrong number of sex chromosomes?

1/500 live births!

Eighty percent of the infants with the wrong number of sex chromosomes have what two errors?

XXX or XYY

(It is more common to have three chromosomes, not to be missing one)

The XXY genotype has what eponymic name?

Klinefelter's syndrome

What are the physical characteristics of Klinefelter's syndrome?
(4)

- **Tall**
- **Gynecomastia**
- **Delayed secondary sexual characteristics**
- **Small testes**

Are Klinefelter's patients able to have children of their own?

No

What sperm abnormality do Klinefelter's patients have?

Azoospermia
(They don't make functional sperm)

When extra X chromosomes are present, what determines the amount of phenotypic abnormality?

Increasing numbers of Xs create increasing abnormalities
($\uparrow$ Xs $\rightarrow$ $\uparrow$ problems)

What is the genotype for Turner's syndrome?

45, X

(one sex chromosome missing)

When an individual has many X chromosomes (for example, 49XXXXX), that individual is usually _____?

Mosaic

(Not all cells carry the abnormality)

What are common cardiac abnormalities for Turner's syndrome patients?

1. *Bicuspid aortic valve (50 %)*
2. *Aortic coarctation*

What percentage of Turner's syndrome fetuses are born live?

1 %

(The rest abort spontaneously)

What physical characteristics are typical of Turner's syndrome girls? (5 main ones)	1. **Webbed neck** 2. **Short stature** 3. **Lack of secondary sex characteristics** 4. **Widely spaced nipples** 5. *Hand or foot lymphedema* **(popular as a photo item on the boards!!!)**
Are Turner's syndrome women likely to be mentally retarded?	**No** Mnemonic: Tina Turner is very successful – no MR there! (Ike, on the other hand … just kidding)
What are the characteristic facial features of Turner's syndrome?	**"Posteriorly rotated" ears** **&** **Triangle face**
Is Turner's syndrome associated with advanced maternal age?	**No –** **It's a missing chromosome syndrome** (not an extra one that stayed stuck together because the two chromosomes had been together for too long!)
When are Turner's syndrome patients most likely to have foot or hand lymphedema?	**In infancy** (Look for a photo of a swollen infant hand or foot!)
What is a "chromosomal instability" syndrome?	What it sounds like – The chromosomes break more often than normal (due to repair enzyme defects, etc.)
What is <u>the</u> most important example of a chromosomal instability syndrome?	Xeroderma pigmentosa (sunlight breaks the DNA & it is not repaired)
In addition to xeroderma pigmentosa, what other chromosomal instability disorders are especially important? (3)	1. <u>A</u>taxia-telangiectasia 2. <u>F</u>anconi syndrome 3. <u>B</u>loom syndrome Mnemonic: Think of an emotionally "unstable" <u>AFB</u> whose DNA keeps breaking

Which ethnic group is least likely to have cleft lip/palate?	African-Americans
Which ethnic group is most likely to have cleft lip/palate?	Native Americans
Are most cleft lip/palate cases inherited?	No – Usually sporadic mutations
If a couple's firstborn child has cleft lip/palate, how likely is it that the next child will also have it?	**3–4 %** (the risk is increased, but not by a lot)
What is the main challenge for infants with cleft lip or palate?	**Feeding & airway issues** (depending on the extent of the anomaly)
What infection are cleft lip and palate kids at increased risk to develop?	**Recurrent otitis media** (& persistent effusion)
Generally, what is the time course for repair of cleft lip and palate?	Lip first (<5 months old) Palate between 6 & 12 months
After cleft lip/palate, what is the second most common malformation of the craniofacial area?	External ear problems combined with maxillary &/or mandibular hypoplasia
The combination of jaw hypoplasia & external ear abnormalities is called _____?	**Hemifacial microsomia**
Hemifacial microsomia is mainly important for its associations. What associated problems do these kids often have? **(3)**	**1. Cervical vertebrae (1/3)** **2. Cardiac anomalies** **3. Renal anomalies**
If a boards vignette indicates that a child has ear abnormalities, and asks what further studies are warranted, what should you be thinking of?	**1. Renal ultrasound** **2. Cardiac ultrasound (or other cardiac eval)**

What does "microtia" mean?

Small outer ear

&

blind or missing external auditory meatus

What is anotia?

One or both external ears are missing (external ear aka pinna or auricle)

Any child with ear malformation is at increased risk for renal malformations – whether or not he or she has hemifacial microsomia. What counts as a malformation of the outer ear?

1. **Microtia (small)**
2. **Anotia (missing)**
3. **Canal atresia**

Note: Preauricular tags do not count anymore! (They used to)

Goldenhar syndrome is essentially the same as what descriptively titled disorder?

Hemifacial microsomia

What is the name for the very unusual finding that often occurs in Goldenhar syndrome?

Epibulbar dermoids

(aka epibulbar lipodermoids – same thing)

What on earth is an epibulbar dermoid?

A fibrofatty mass on the globe of the eye – usually inferolateral

If a patient only has epibulbar dermoids as an abnormal finding, what is the diagnosis?

Goldenhar syndrome

(In this case, you wouldn't diagnose hemifacial microsomia, because the rest of the face is normal)

Does Goldenhar syndrome have a particular inheritance pattern?

No –
usually sporadic

What sensory problem do Goldenhar syndrome patients often have?

Conductive hearing loss

There are two important facial anomaly syndromes that have autosomal _dominant_ inheritance patterns. What are they?

1. **BOR syndrome (Branchiootorenal (BOR))**
2. **Treacher–Collins**

What are the problems for BOR syndrome?

1. Branchial area – fistulas, cysts, preauricular pits
2. Oto – cochlear & stapes malformations, plus hearing problems
3. Renal – dysplasia & aplasia

How is BOR syndrome inherited?

AD
(Autosomal dominant)

How can you remember BOR syndrome?

Wild <u>BO</u>ARS are aggressive & *dominant*

This particular one is dancing around because he needs to pee, but can't (no kidneys). He has an ugly, lumpy neck (fistulas & cysts) and won't come when he's called! (Can't hear)

Treacher–Collins syndrome is very similar to hemifacial microsomia, except that it involves what two other structures?

Zygoma (cheek bone)

&

Eyes (usually colobomata of the lower lid)

FYI: Colobomas are a failure of the two sides of the iris/uveal layer of the eye to fuse at the bottom Looks like a cleft at the bottom of the iris

Is craniosynostosis usually an inherited or a sporadic disorder?

Sporadic

What is craniosynostosis?

Abnormally early fusion of the skull sutures
(usually just some of them)

Why is craniosynostosis a bad thing?
(3)

1. **Risk of ↑ ICP**
2. **Creates facial abnormalities**
3. **Creates an odd head shape**

Which cranial suture is most often involved in craniosynostosis?

The sagittal suture

(the one that runs down the middle of the skull, dividing it into left & right sides)

Is sagittal synostosis more common in males or females?

Males
(5:1)

What head shape develops with sagittal craniosynostosis?

Long & narrow – like a boat

("scaphocephaly" aka "dolichocephaly")

Where is the coronal suture?

Goes from ear to ear, like a girl's headband!

Unilateral coronal or sphenofrontal suture fusion leads to what facial abnormalities?
                        (3)

1. **Flattened forehead**
2. **High orbit & eyebrow**
3. **Prominent ear**
(**all unilateral on the affected side**)

What is the other name for the triad of flat (unilateral) forehead, elevated eye, & prominent ear, in addition to "coronal & sphenofrontal craniosynostosis?"

Frontal plagiocephaly

When the coronal & sphenofrontal sutures are bilaterally involved in craniosynostosis, what head shape will result?

Cone head
(**officially "turricephaly"**)

Mnemonic:
Think of how a "turret" sticks up on a tank or a building to remember that "turret-cephaly" is a sticking up cone head

Where is the "metopic" suture?

It's the vertical suture in the middle of the forehead

Metopic suture craniosynostosis results in what forehead shape?

"Keel shaped"
(**like the keel of a boat – coming to a point or a ridge**)

Metopic craniosynostosis results in what overall head shape?

Triangular
(**officially, "trigonocephaly" – like the shape of one of those "three-cornered" hats popular during the American revolution!**)

Does craniosynostosis require treatment?

Yes

What treatment is recommended for craniosynostosis, and why?

- **Surgery**
- **Cosmesis & to remove the risk of ICP issues**

If a patient has craniosynostosis, when is the optimum time for surgical correction?

Before the point of most rapid head growth
(<5 months is ideal)

Frontal plagiocephaly is more common in which gender?

Females
(unlike sagittal, which is more common in males)

Where is the lamboid suture?

Back of the head – lower part

Isolated craniosynostosis of the lamboid suture is very uncommon. What changes to head shape will it create?

Flat occipitoparietal area

Lamboid craniosynostosis presents similarly to what far more common head malformation?

Plagiocephaly
(non-pathological flattening due to sleep positioning)

On the board exam, which is more likely – positional plagiocephaly or isolated lamboid craniosynostosis?

Positional plagiocephaly!!!

Does positional plagiocephaly require treatment?

No
(Severe cases can be given a sleeping helmet – rarely needed, though)

If you are not certain whether your patient has lamboid synostosis or plagiocephaly, what test will differentiate them?

CT of the skull –
synostosis will have sclerotic connection of the lamboid suture

When will plagiocephaly stop progressing (on its own)?

7 months

When will lamboid synostosis stop progressing?

It won't
(without intervention)

What physical findings suggest plagio-cephaly, rather than lamboid craniosynostosis?

1. Ear goes <u>anterior</u>
2. Frontal prominence
3. Lack of any posterior prominence (often unilateral effects in both conditions)

Plagiocephaly is often associated with what other disorder?

Torticollis
(makes sense – they *can't* turn their heads)

What is the name of the most common skeletal dysplasia?

Achondroplasia

What are the two essential skeletal differences seen with achondroplasia?

Short stature

&

"Rhizomelic shortening"

What is rhizomelic shortening?

The proximal parts of the limbs are more shortened than the distal portions

(For example, the upper arm is especially short, compared to the lower arm)

What are the characteristic facial features of achondroplastic individuals?
(3)

Prominent forehead
Flat nasal bridge
Mid-face hypoplasia

Are the heads of achondroplastic patients unusually large or small?

Large
(macrocephaly)

Does achondroplasia affect intelligence?

No
(Think of all of the successful achondroplastic actors!)

When achondroplasia is inherited, what is the inheritance pattern?

Autosomal dominant

If two achondroplastic adults decide to have a child, what are the possible outcomes for the child, and how likely is each?

Homozygous – fatal – 25 %
No bad genes – normal – 25 %
Heterozygous – affected – 50 %

Are most cases of achondroplasia inherited?	**No –** **Most are new mutations**
What risk factor increases the probability of a child having achondroplasia due to a new mutation?	**Advanced paternal age**
What is the buzzword for the appearance of the hand in achondroplasia?	**"Trident" hands** **(short hand with broad fingers – normal number, though!)**
Are there often other (organ) abnormalities associated with achondroplasia?	No
Are achondroplastic children easily identified at birth?	No – But they fall to 5 % in length in the first 3 months of life
What is the usual final height of achondroplastic patients?	3–4 ft
What serious set of complications sometimes develops during infancy for achondroplastic patients?	**Foramen magnum stenosis** **&/or** **craniocervical junction abnormalities**
What problems can result from achondroplastic abnormalities of the craniocervical junction & foramen magnum? **(4)**	**Apnea** **Hydrocephalus** **Paralysis** **Growth delay**
What unusual health maintenance is recommended for achondroplastic patients during infancy?	**Monthly monitoring of head circumference** **(& careful measurement of the size & shape of fontanelle)**
What common infection are achondroplasia kids especially likely to develop?	Serous otitis media
How is the achondroplasia diagnosis confirmed?	Usually X-ray

What hip & pelvis X-ray findings are considered to be typical for achondroplasia?	1. **Thick femoral necks** 2. **"Ice cream scoop-shaped" femoral heads** 3. **Squared off iliac wings** 4. **Flat or irregular acetabular roof**
The single amino acid substitution involved in achondroplasia has what consequences for bone development? (2)	1. Decreased chrondrocytes & ↓ bone matrix production 2. Decreased ossification of growing bone matrix
Fibroblast growth factor receptor 3 (FGFR3) is the gene responsible for what two groups of skeletal dysplasias?	1. Achondroplasia 2. Thanatophoric dysplasias (almost always lethal) (thanatos – Greek name for the guy in the big cloak who represents death!)
The FGFR3 gene is located on which chromosome?	4p
There are two types of thanatophoric dysplasias – I & II. Which one has a "clover leaf" skull?	II Mnemonic: Think of there being two sides to the clover leaf
Both types of thanatophoric dysplasias have what typical characteristics?	1. Big head 2. Short limbs 3. Flat vertebral bodies (platyspondyly)
The special finding that identifies a type II thanatophoric dysplasia patient is _____?	**Cloverleaf skull**
Platyspondyly, meaning flattened vertebral bodies, is a characteristic of what disorder?	Thanatophoric dysplasias (both types)
Which type of osteogenesis imperfecta keeps their blue sclerae throughout the life-span?	**Type 1**
There are four types of osteogenesis imperfecta. Which is the most common?	**Type 1** **(It is also the mildest)**

There are two relatively mild forms of osteogenesis imperfecta. What are they?

Type 1 (most common)

&

Type 4

One aspect of their presentation often allows us to distinguish types 1 & 4 osteogenesis at birth. What is it?

Birth fractures are *common* with type 4, but *rare* in type 1

Which type of osteogenesis is the mildest, if you must choose only one?

Type 1 (most common & mildest)

When do type 1 osteogenesis patients develop most of their fractures?

Childhood (fewer fractures in adolescence)

In addition to the likelihood of birth fractures, what other factors distinguish type 1 osteogenesis from type 4?

- **Blue sclerae throughout the life-span (type 4 have white)**

- **Normal height (type 4 are short)**

Which type of osteogenesis imperfecta starts with blue sclerae but lightens to white or near-white in time?

Type 3 (Short patients – often can't ambulate)

Osteogenesis imperfecta types I & IV share their mild manifestations, and what tooth problem?

Dentinogenesis imperfecta (pearly looking teeth with enamel that flakes off easily)

Can dentinogenesis imperfecta occur in patients who *do not* have osteogenesis imperfecta?

Yes – It can also be an isolated autosomal dominant disorder

A *short patient* with *white sclerae* presents to your office. The child has a history of *two fractures at birth, and the lower legs are bowed out*. Which type of osteogenesis imperfecta is this likely to be?

Type 4

For type 1 osteogenesis imperfecta patients, what complications often occur in their 20s & 30s?
(2)

1. Scoliosis
2. Hearing loss

What is the underlying problem in osteogenesis imperfecta type 1?

Decreased type 1 collagen

What are the typical characteristics of an osteogenesis imperfecta type 1 patient?

(5)

1. **Blue sclerae**
2. **Multiple <u>childhood</u> fractures**
3. **Normal or near-normal height**
4. **Lax joints**
5. **Mild osteopenia on X-ray**

What is abnormal about the fontanelles in osteogenesis patients?

Delayed closure

Which type of osteogenesis imperfecta is the most severe, usually causing death within *a few weeks*?

Type 2
(death due to respiratory insufficiency)

The X-ray appearance of the bones in osteogenesis type II features what two unusual findings?

1. "Beading" of the ribs (due to many calluses along their length)
2. "Crumpled appearance" of the long bones

The mild cases of osteogenesis usually have mutations of which gene?
What about the severe types?

• COLIA1

• COLIA1 or COLIA2

What are the classic eye findings for type IV osteogenesis imperfecta?

White or near-white

When osteogenesis imperfecta is transmitted as an inherited disease (rather than as a new mutation), what is the usual inheritance pattern?

Autosomal dominant

(there are some autosomal recessive cases, but these are much less common)

Type IV osteogenesis is mild but still often has fractures present at birth. What is the <u>hallmark</u> of type IV?

"Tibial bowing"

Describe the classic type IV patient?

1. Short stature
2. Tibial bowing
3. Birth fractures
4. White sclerae
5. Bad teeth
(dentinogenesis imperfecta)

Are severe forms of a disease that presents in childhood usually inherited or new mutations (assuming that the disease would have an autosomal dominant inheritance pattern)?

New mutations

(Because a severely affected individual would have to reproduce in order to pass a dominant disorder, which is not likely!)

Neurological complications of osteogenesis imperfecta are most common in which type?

Type 3

What types of neurological complications are often seen with type 3 osteogenesis?

Hydrocephalus
&
"Basilar skull invagination"

Patients with which type of osteogenesis often survive but may not be able to ambulate due to frequent fractures?

Type 3

(Fractures due to supporting their own weight!!)

What is especially unusual about the eye findings in osteogenesis type 3?

Sclerae are blue at birth but lighten with age

Problems with which organ system result in the most deaths for Marfan's patients?

Cardiovascular

How is Marfan's inherited?

Autosomal dominant

How can you quickly differentiate Marfan's from homocystinuria, a disorder with which it shares many features?
(Lab test)

Check urine for homocystine (elevated in homocystinuria)

The urine test for homocystinuria should be done when the patient is not taking significant supplements of _____?

Pyridoxine! (vitamin B$_6$)

(Can cause a false negative)

Homocystinuria & Marfan's present differently on physical exam. Which one has a downwardly dislocated eye lens and mental retardation?

Homocystinuria
(the lens goes down like the IQ)

Tipoffs the board likes to give for Marfan's syndrome are _____?

1. **High arched palate**
2. *Dislocated lens (UP)*
3. **Mitral valve prolapse**
4. **Pectus carinatum/excavatum**

What is pectus carinatum & pectus excavatum?

- **Carinatum sticks out like a pigeon's chest**
- **Excavatum goes in (like an excavation)**

What is another way to say "dislocated lens?"

Ectopia lentis

Which gene is often responsible for Marfan's syndrome?

Fibrillin 1 (FBN 1)

If you suspect the Marfan's diagnosis, and a patient has an affected first-degree relative, what additional findings must be present to confirm the diagnosis?

Ectopia lentis OR
Aortic root dilatation OR
Systemic score ≥7

If you suspect a patient has Marfan's, but there are no affected relatives, what is required to make the diagnosis?
   (3 options)

Aortic root dilatation +
Ectopic lentis OR systemic score ≥7
(similar to above)

OR

Aortic root dilatation + presence of FBN1 mutation

OR

Ectopia lentis + FBN1 mutation + history of previous aortic disease

What cardiovascular complications, in particular, are common among Marfan's patients?

Aortic dissection/rupture/ dilation

What medications are helpful in managing Marfan's?

β-blockers (to slow aortic dilatation)

Is all exercise bad in Marfan's syndrome patients?

No –
Aerobic, gentle exercise is good

What types of exercise are dangerous for Marfan's patients?

Exercise that raises the blood pressure significantly or suddenly (NO weight lifting!)

Why is early induction of puberty sometimes recommended for Marfan's patients?

To limit height & kyphoscoliosis

What special risk do Marfan's patients face, if they become pregnant?

Accelerated aortic dilation

What foot abnormality do Marfan's patients often have?

Flat foot
(pes planus, officially)

What is "thumb sign" in Marfan's syndrome?

The thumb goes beyond the border of the hand, when folded across the palm

What is "wrist sign" in Marfan's syndrome?

The thumb & fifth finger overlap, when wrapped around the wrist

(present on a lot of normal folks, too)

What skin finding is sometimes seen in Marfan's syndrome?

**Striae atrophica
("stretch marks" on the belly, buttocks, & thighs)**

(a minor criterion)

What pulmonary issues are more common in Marfan's patients?

(Apical) blebs & pneumothoraces

Is it alright for Ehlers–Danlos patients to play contact sports? Why or why not?

No –
Danger to joints

&

skin splits very easily!
  (yuck)

**What is the classic Ehlers–Danlos syndrome?
(Four attributes)**

1. **Hyperextensible skin**
2. **Hypermobile joints**
3. **Easy bruising**
4. **Dystrophic scarring**

Why do Ehlers–Danlos patients bruise easily?

"Capillary fragility" is abnormal

(other bleeding parameters are fine)

How many types of Ehlers–Danlos are there?

Seven major variants –
so signs can vary from patient to patient

What unusual health maintenance is needed for Marfan's syndrome patients?

**Routine echocardiogram
Q6–12 months
(to monitor the aorta, mainly)**

In Ehlers–Danlos, how is the skin usually described?

• Spongy, stretchy
• Returns to original appearance after stretching (snaps back)
• Extra skin is often present

Are the large or the small joints affected in Ehlers–Danlos?	Both (Dislocations are also common)
What is the main intervention possible with Ehlers–Danlos patients?	Protect the skin with shin guards, knee pads, etc.
Neurofibromatosis type 1 classically consists of what two findings?	**Cutaneous neurofibromas** **&** **Café-au-lait spots**
At what age can an NF type 1 diagnosis usually be made?	10 years
What are neurofibromas?	Benign Schwann cell & fibroblast growths
In addition to café-au-lait spots, what other easily identifiable findings are common in NF 1? (2)	Iris hamartomas (known as "Lisch nodules") & Axillary freckling
What is usually the earliest sign of NF1?	**Café-au-lait spots** **(<2 years old)**
Are café-au-lait spots unique to NF1?	**No** **(e.g., McCune–Albright has them)**
What percentage of NF1 patients will have axillary freckles or Lisch nodules by puberty?	**75 %**
How is NF1 inherited?	**Autosomal dominant**
What percentage of NF1 cases are actually new mutations, rather than inherited diseases?	**60 %**
Neurofibromatosis type 1 is a neurocutaneous disorder, so it should affect the nervous system & skin. What other system is usually affected?	Bones – Long bone bowing, scoliosis, etc.

In addition to the neurofibromas, themselves, how else does the disorder affect the nervous system?	Learning disabilities Speech impediments Headaches Constipation
Is the genetic cause of neurofibromatosis type 1 related to that of NF2?	No
What causes NF1?	Defective neurofibromin gene (Chromosome 17)
What causes NF2?	Chromosome 22 mutation
How consistent should you expect the manifestations of NF1 to be, across affected family members?	Quite variable (Variable penetrance)
What is the hallmark of NF2?	**Bilateral acoustic neuromas**
If one family member is diagnosed with NF2, what should you do for the other family members?	**MRI screening for acoustic neuromas small enough to remove & preserve hearing**
What is one of the earliest signs of NF2?	Lens opacities/cataracts
What is the other name for an acoustic neuroma?	**Vestibular schwannoma**
What proportion of NF2 patients has tumors other than acoustic neuromas?	50 %
What symptoms do acoustic neuromas cause?	**Hearing loss** **Tinnitus** **Balance problems** **Facial weakness** (Makes sense: The tumor affects CN 8 – vestibulocochlear nerve)
Where do acoustic neuromas usually grow?	CPA – the Cerebellopontine angle
What other tumors (in addition to acoustic neuromas) are common in NF2? (4)	1. Meningiomas 2. Ependymomas Other schwannomas: 3. Spinal schwannomas 4. Schwannomas of other cranial nerves

More than half the time you see an NF1 patient, the disorder occurred due to _____?	New mutation
What eye tumor are NF1 patients at especially high risk to develop?	Optic glioma
Disorders with axillary freckling, such as NF1, often also have freckles on what part of the body?	Groin
What are the two most classic skin findings for tuberous sclerosis?	Ash-leaf spots (hypopigmented) & Shagreen patches (oval plaques on trunk or back)
In addition to ash-leaf spots & shagreen patches, what other skin & nail findings are often seen in tuberous sclerosis? (3)	1. Facial angiomas 2. Forehead plaques (light or yellow) 3. Nail & gingival fibromas
Infants with tuberous sclerosis often have what type of cardiac tumor (50 %)?	Cardiac rhabdomyoma
What unusual diagnostic can help you diagnose the ash-leaf spots of tuberous sclerosis?	They enhance with a Wood's lamp
What are the two main management issues for children with tuberous sclerosis?	Cardiac arrhythmias (due to rhabdomyomas) & Seizures
What is the particular type of seizure activity common in tuberous sclerosis?	Infantile spasm
If an infant has an infantile spasm, what is the likelihood that the child has tuberous sclerosis?	50 %

Which medication is recommended for treatment of the infantile spasms that often accompany tuberous sclerosis?	Vigabatrin
How consistent are the findings of tuberous sclerosis, across affected family members?	Not consistent (variable penetrance)
What is the usual fate for tuberous sclerosis patients with cardiac rhabdomyomas?	They regress by adulthood (as do some of the other usual findings)
What is the main problem in von Hippel–Landau syndrome?	**Multisystem cancers – including hemangioblastomas (usually cerebellar)**
What is the largest cause of death for von Hippel–Landau patients?	**Renal cell cancer (usually in 40s)**
What are the two most common presentations of von Hippel–Landau?	1. **Cerebellar hemangioblastomas in an adolescent** 2. **Retinal angioma in childhood**
What causes von Hippel–Landau syndrome?	Loss of a tumor-suppressor gene on chromosome 3 (the "VHL" tumor-suppressor gene) (VHL stands for von Hippel–Landau)
Are the tumors of von Hippel–Landau syndrome benign or malignant?	Both
Which organs most commonly develop tumors in von Hippel–Landau? (5)	1. **CNS (esp. cerebellum)** 2. **Neuroendocrine tissue (e.g., adrenals & pheochromocytoma)** 3. **Retina** 4. **Pancreas** 5. **Kidney**
The most classic tumor, histologically speaking, in von Hippel–Landau is _____?	**Hemangioblastoma**

Tuberous sclerosis & the NF disorders have a lot of variation in their penetrance. What about von Hippel–Landau?

It is highly penetrant (and autosomal dominant!)

Poor development of the cheek bones, cleft palate, small chin, and missing lashes on the lower medial eyelid = _____?

Treacher–Collins syndrome (a craniofacial syndrome)

Most craniofacial syndromes have what type of inheritance pattern?

Autosomal dominant

If a craniofacial syndrome is not autosomal dominant in its inheritance, it is likely to be _____?

Sporadic mutation

Partial albinism, premature gray hair, and a *white forelock* of hair are tipoffs to which craniofacial syndrome?

Waardenburg

In addition to "hair" findings, what else do you expect in Waardenburg's syndrome?

1. Cleft lip/palate
2. Eye findings
(iris heterochromia & telecanthus)

What is telecanthus?

Wide-set eyes

Sturge–Weber patients often have what visible manifestation of their disorder?

Capillary malformations in the trigeminal distribution (meningeal hemangiomata are hidden beneath!)

What chronic clinical problem do Sturge–Weber patients often suffer from?

Seizures

Is Sturge–Weber typically inherited or sporadic?

Sporadic

Cone head (turricephaly) due to craniosynostosis, proptosis, & maxillary hypoplasia are the major characteristics of which craniofacial disorder?

Crouzon syndrome

Craniosynostosis with proptosis, broad thumbs, and fusion of digits 2, 3, & 4 suggests what diagnosis?

Apert syndrome

Mnemonic:
Think of someone wearing an apron with broad thumbs tucked inside the pocket and fused fingers on the outside. The baker is shocked that her food is burning, so her eyes are "bugging out," and her mouth is open in a big "O," showing her high palate!

A "cathedral ceiling" narrow palate is a buzzword for what *craniofacial* syndrome?

Apert syndrome

Crouzon syndrome & Apert syndrome are fairly similar. What is one easy way to distinguish them?

Apert has syndactyly (remember the hands in the apron) – Crouzon does not

High arched palate in the setting of a connective tissue disorder = what diagnosis?

Marfan's syndrome

The main characteristics in Crouzon syndrome are _____?
(3)

1. Turricephaly due to craniosynostosis (cone head)
2. Proptosis (& some other eye findings)
3. Maxillary hypoplasia

Delayed eruption of both permanent & deciduous teeth, along with other tooth abnormalities such as extra teeth & fused teeth, are characteristics of what craniofacial disorder?

Cleidocranial dysostosis

In addition to tooth abnormalities, cleidocranial dysostosis patients may also have abnormalities of the skull & what two other structures?

Clavicles (missing or hypoplastic)

&

Lax joints

A baker is wearing an *apron*. She is shocked that her food is burning, so her eyes are bugging out and her mouth is open in a big "O" showing a high, arched palate. She has broad thumbs tucked into her apron, with syndactylous fingers on the outside. Which disorder is this?

Apert syndrome

Frequent infections, malignancies, ataxia, and telangiectasias describe what recessive disorder?

Ataxia telangiectasia

Pancytopenia, *hypoplastic thumb & radius*, dark pigmentation, & facial abnormalities =

Fanconi anemia

Facial telangiectasias + everything small (microcephaly, IUGR, & malar hypoplasia) =

Bloom syndrome

Mnemonic:
Think of the patient's facial telangiectasias as "blooms" on a very small face

Bloom syndrome patients are also at risk for what problematic complication?

Malignancies

The hallmarks of Apert syndrome are _____?

(3)

1. Broad thumbs, often with digits 2, 3, & 4 fused
2. Proptosis
3. Craniosynostosis

If a vignette mentions *cysteine crystals in the cornea*, what syndrome is the correct diagnosis?

Nephropathic cystinosis

(They also have Fanconi syndrome)

Big tongue, big head, and coarse facies should make you think of what congenital syndrome?

Beckwith–Wiedemann

What special ear finding is classic for Beckwith–Wiedemann?

Earlobe "fissures" or crease

What abdominal abnormality is common in Beckwith–Wiedemann?

Omphalocele

Which tumors are Beckwith–Wiedemann patients at risk to develop?

Wilms & testicular (due to cryptorchidism)

Are there any special health maintenance protocols for Beckwith–Wiedemann patients?

Yes –
Serial abdominal US every 3 months until 8 years old (Wilms tumor)

&

Serial AFPs until 4 years old (also Wilms tumor)

What causes Beckwith–Wiedemann?

Paternal uniparental disomy (11p15.5)

Short children with very little hair & eczema probably have what syndrome?

Dubowitz syndrome

How is the face of a Dubowitz syndrome patient unusual?

Telecanthus
Eczema
Droopy lids (ptosis)
Not much hair

(Think of a little kid named "TED" Dubowitz, who doesn't have much hair)

What is unusual about the face of a *Williams syndrome* patient?

Upturned nares

&

Stellate iris

Pectus excavatum, webbed neck, and wide-set eyes on a short patient suggests what congenital disorder?

Noonan syndrome

Noonan patients have pectus excavatum. What cardiovascular abnormality do they have?

Pulmonary valve stenosis is most common

(Think of the stenosis as choking off the blood supply to the chest – making it sink in)

What circulatory issues are common in Noonan syndrome patients?

Lymphedema

&

Bleeding diathesis

Are you likely to see Noonan syndrome in men or women?

Both –
More common in men, though

A child with sensorineural deafness most often has what very general, underlying cause?

Genetic disorders

Is history of pyloric stenosis in the mother or the father most predictive of whether children will be born with pyloric stenosis?

**Maternal history
(but boys more often affected, overall)**

If two children with cleft lip or palate have been born to the same couple, what does this mean for the probability of recurrence?

It doubles

At what point in development can amniocentesis sampling for genetic disorders be done?

16 weeks

(& results often take at least 1 week to be ready)

(Chorionic villus sampling can be done after 10 weeks)

Craniosynostosis & syndactyly occurring together is most often what genetic syndrome?

Apert syndrome

Do CHARGE syndrome patients have normal intelligence?

No –
Think of it as a patient with an uncontrollable shopping habit. They've "charged away" all their intelligence!

What problems do CHARGE patients have?

Coloboma
Heart disease
Atresia (choanal)
Retarded growth
Genital/GU anomalies
Ear anomalies

In an X-linked <u>dominant</u> disorder, what unique inheritance pattern do you expect between father & their children?

<u>All</u> females are affected, & no males

(affected mothers pass it on to 50 % of all children)

What are the basics of the progeria genetic disease?

Premature aging

&

Very-early-onset atherosclerosis

How is progeria different from Cockayne syndrome?

Both look like little old people, but – Cockayne adds eye problems and photosensitive skin

How can you remember the main features of Cockayne syndrome?

Picture an old "Cockney" guy wearing dark glasses due to his eye problems, who is desperate to get into the pub – to get his photosensitive skin out of the sun (and get his beer)!

What are the components of Holt–Oram syndrome?

1. Three-jointed thumb (often)
2. Arm defects
3. ASD
Mnemonic:
It's hard to "hold your arm (Holt–Oram)" with a three-jointed thumb!

A short male adolescent presents with lymphedema, and on physical exam you notice a webbed neck, pectus excavatum, and a systolic murmur. Which disorder is this?

Noonan syndrome

(pulmonary valve stenosis is common)

Which age group of women most commonly gives birth to Down syndrome children?

Women in their 20s

(Why? They have more babies, and they are less often tested for Down's fetuses.)

Genetic translocations, rather than a full extra copy of chromosome 21, account for what percentage of Down's cases?

About 5 %

Are the phenotypic features of Down syndrome different for children with trisomy vs. translocation?

No

Is it important to identify the reason Down's has occurred?
(e.g., trisomy vs. translocation)

Yes –
Important to prediction of future risk

(Recurrence risk with trisomy is 1 % in women without advanced maternal age, but it is higher if there is a translocation)

Which Down's translocation causes a very high likelihood of recurrence?

Full 21q translocation
(21q21q)

How can you remember that Treacher–Collins syndrome patients have normal intelligence?

You can't have MR and still be a t(r) eacher!

How can you remember that Treacher–Collins is an autosomal dominant disorder?

Think of a very bossy (dominant) teacher, with an unruly class!

Since Treacher–Collins is an AD disorder, family information that might help you make the diagnosis includes what two scenarios?

A family photo showing multiple family members with:
1. **Small chins & lower lid problems**
2. *Hearing aids*

Café-au-lait skin spots, plus abnormal bones & a child going through early puberty = what syndrome?

McCune–Albright

How can you remember that VATER or VACTERL patients generally have normal intelligence?

VATER is close to the word "father," like a priest. To get through training to be a priest (father) you'd need good intelligence

At birth, how do VACTERL patients often first come to medical attention?

Single umbilical artery!!!

If an infant has a single umbilical artery, what structural anomaly is especially likely?

Renal anomalies

"Punched out" scalp lesions – meaning portions of the scalp that are not covered with skin – go with which trisomy?

Unlucky 13!

Trisomy 13 has the bad luck number in its name. How can you remember the attributes of trisomy 13?

13 fingers sticking into the holes in the head, including the holes made by a cleft lip & palate

Where the fingers are stuck in, they get abscesses – due to faulty PMNs

When they stick the *13 fingers* into their belly, *two hit the ovaries*, damaging them (hypoplastic)
Two hit the uterus, making it bicornuate (meaning there are two separated parts to the uterus)
The remaining nine hit the kidneys, leaving them with cystic kidneys

How can you remember the set of abnormalities that goes with trisomy 18?

Think of an 18-year-old "angry young man" with his *fist clenched* so hard his *nails become hypoplastic*

He rocks back and forth on *rocker bottom feet* in frustration, after banging his head against the wall of society's expectations (*big occiput*)

His attitude isn't the only thing bent out of shape – so are his kidneys! They're horseshoe shaped

Should parents have genetic testing anytime they give birth to a child with a trisomy?

<u>Yes</u> –
Birth of <u>any trisomy</u> increases the risk of having another child with various anomalies

Which relatively common hematological disorders can be diagnosed prenatally?

Factors 8 & 9 deficiency

&

Sickle cell

A child with seizures, mental retardation, and history significant for infantile spasms has what genetic disorder?

Tuberous sclerosis

How can you remember the underlying genetic issue in Cri-du-chat syndrome? (Just checking whether you remembered!)

If cats are supposed to have nine lives, then these kids have used up <u>5</u> of them just making it to the delivery room!

(Cats are small animals, so you know it must be the "p" part of the chromosome: 5p-)

If a vignette tells you that a Down syndrome patient needs a sports physical because he or she wishes to participate in Special Olympics, what should you be concerned about?

Atlanto-axial instability

If a vignette features a Down syndrome kid with a neurological complaint, what should your first thought be?

Atlanto-axial instability might be the cause

What unusual torso finding sometimes occurs in Down syndrome?

12th rib missing

Mnemonic:
12 is 21 backwards

What are the main features of Crouzon syndrome, and how can you remember them?

Prominent eyes and forehead (due to craniosynostosis), with receding chin

Mnemonic:
The shape of the head makes them "aerodynamic for cruisin' in a convertible!"

How can you remember the inheritance pattern of Crouzon syndrome?

Kids that go out cruisin' are <u>dominant</u> & popular, compared to the ones who stay home

(+ nearly all craniofacial syndromes are dominant)

Microcephaly, seizures, eye problems, and a <u>missing corpus callosum</u> go with what syndrome?

Aicardi

Mnemonic:
Think of a-corp-i, meaning "without corpi" or without corpus callosum

What is very unusual about the inheritance of Aicardi syndrome?

It is X-linked <u>dominant</u>

(like incontinentia pigmenti – the skin disorder)

How can you remember the critical ingredients of "Rubinstein–Taybi" syndrome?

The thumb's base is broad, but the scrotum's base is small – because it's hanging empty due to cryptorchidism!

Think of the broad-based thumb looped around the narrow-based, empty, scrotum

What abnormality gives Russell–Silver syndrome patients a "triangular" face?

Micrognathia

Russell–Silver sounds like "Russell Stover" – the candy company. How can this help you to remember the problems Russell–Silver patients have?

If you only ate candy, you would be *growth retarded* and you might have a small jaw due to the candy rotting it away
(They don't have tooth problems, though, just micrognathia)

If a vignette describes a tall male patient with normal intelligence, but who is "socially awkward," what syndrome might they be hinting at?	Klinefelter's (47 XXY)
How can you remember that Klinefelter's patients have small testes?	"Kleine" means small in Dutch/ German and is spelled nearly the same
Why is it important to do chromosomal screening on Turner's syndrome patients?	**Because they often have a partial Y chromosome – this puts them at risk for gonadoblastoma**
Diseases that are inherited exclusively through the mother are usually due to _____?	**Mitochondrial inheritance** (genomic imprinting is also a possibility)
If a disorder can result from more than one genetic error (such as Tay–Sachs), it is said to have _____ _____.	**Genetic heterogeneity**
Homeobox or HOX genes are important in what aspect of development?	Early differentiation (in the embryo) into tissues & body segments
Are homeobox gene mutations known to produce genetic syndromes in humans?	Yes – Waardenburg & others
PCR is a technique used in genetic research to do what?	Greatly increase the amount of DNA or RNA available for evaluation ("amplifying" it)
Genetic "anticipation" refers to what pattern in inherited diseases?	**Worsening severity as the generations progress**
In a disorder with multifactorial inheritance, the more severely the patient is affected, the _____ the likelihood of his/her children being affected.	Greater (Presumably, more genes were present, producing the more severe manifestations and increasing the probability that at least some of the genes will be passed on)
How high will the concordance rate be for twins in a family affected by a multifactorial disorder?	Variable (usually 20–65 %)

In multifactorial disorders, are there symptomatic carriers?

No –
You are either affected or not

Can a translocation of chromosome 21 to a different chromosome still cause Down syndrome?

Yes
(Common Down's translocations involve chromosomes 21, 13, 14, & 15)

If a gonadal tumor develops in a Turner's syndrome patient, what is the likely cause?

The patient had some portion of the Y chromosome

Hypomelanosis of Ito is usually a mosaic disorder (not all body cells carry the abnormality). How can you test for it?

Do chromosome studies on skin fibroblasts
(lymphocyte studies are often negative)

What are the main features of hypomelanosis of Ito?

1. **Macules of hypopigmented areas – in streaks & whorls**
2. **Ocular problems**
3. **CNS problems**

The FISH technique enables identification of what?

The <u>chromosomal location</u> of a particular gene

A patient presents with a recessive disorder. Neither parent has the disorder. Chromosome testing of the parents shows that only one of them carries the gene. How is this possible?

Uniparental isodisomy
(from Mom)

What is uniparental disomy?

A complicated genetic goof up –
One parent contributes both copies of a gene for something

A newborn infant who was born *breech*, with a history of *polyhydramnios*, is noted to have *hypotonia, flat face & occiput*, and a *distended abdomen*. What is the most likely diagnosis?

Trisomy 21
(the polyhydramnios & distended abdomen are probably due to duodenal atresia)

Hemihypertrophy with soft tissue growth like the "Elephant Man," big fingers, and skin nevi go with what disorder?

Proteus syndrome

How did Proteus syndrome get its name?

So many different things are growing/ happening in the disorder –
There are "protean" (meaning many) effects

A large-for-gestation-age infant (LGA) with big hands, feet, & head who is also mentally retarded has what syndrome?

Sotos syndrome

(The lateral eye margins also look as if they are sloping downward – Actress Katie Holmes has eyes with this feature)

How can you remember the features of Sotos syndrome?

Think of a baby with everything "big at the ends"
(hands, feet, head – even the "toes," as in So – toes!)

What is the Poland anomaly?

Pectoralis major & minor are missing

Mnemonic:
In WWII, the Russian invasion of Poland effectively "cut off the country's right arm" in its attempt to defend itself. Poland anomaly is missing the muscles needed to control (either) arm

Poland anomaly, along with ipsilateral breast hypoplasia and missing rib segments, limb abnormalities, and cranial nerve problems, goes with what genetic syndrome?

Moebius syndrome

How can you remember Moebius syndrome?

Think of one arm, with its associated muscles and nearby structures, replaced by a Mobius strip

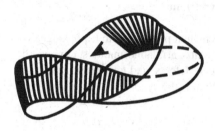

Is there any special inheritance pattern for Moebius syndrome?

No –
It's sporadic

What does "TAR," as in TAR syndrome, stand for?

Thrombocytopenia
Absent
Radius syndrome

In TAR syndrome, are the radii usually missing on one side or both sides?

Both sides

Problems with the "radial ray," which forms the radius & thumbs, often co-occur with problems in what other system?

The blood
(Anemia, thrombocytopenia, pancytopenia)

In TAR syndrome, are the thumbs abnormal?

NO!

Congenital heart defects, triphalangeal thumb, and other radial ray abnormalities go with what two syndromes?

Holt–Oram
&
Diamond–Blackfan

How can you distinguish the two syndromes that involved triphalangeal thumbs, radial ray defects, and congenital heart abnormalities?

Diamond–Blackfan also has hypoplastic anemia

(This is rare with Holt–Oram)

A patient with triphalangeal thumb, arm abnormalities, and an ASD is likely to have what congenital syndrome?

Holt–Oram
(no blood abnormalities)

An infant is born without radii bilaterally, but the thumbs are normal. Routine lab work shows thrombocytopenia. What is the syndrome?

TAR
(Thrombocytopenia – absent radius)

A patient presents with triphalangeal thumbs, arm abnormalities, congenital heart defects, and *hypoplastic anemia*. What is the syndrome?

Diamond–Blackfan
(They should have called it "white fan" because the patients are so anemic they'll look white – not black!)

A dark (hyperpigmented) child with hypoplastic thumbs & radii, pancytopenia, and a funny face has what congenital syndrome?

Fanconi's anemia

Mnemonic:
Mispronounce
Fan-co-ni like <u>Pan</u>-co-ni to remind yourself that they have <u>pan</u>cytopenia

<u>Tan</u>-co-ni reminds you that they can be hyperpigmented

How is Beckwith–Wiedemann syndrome inherited?

Autosomal dominant

Mnemonic:
Everything is so big in Beckwith–Wiedemann, it's got to be dominant!

One side of the body larger than the other, sporadic inheritance, skin marks (nevi & hemangiomata), and soft tissue "lumps" means what syndrome?

Proteus
(The Elephant Man – many or "protean" growths)

Meckel–Gruber syndrome is lethal. It features microcephaly with what occipital malformation?

Encephalocele

In addition to CNS issues with microcephaly & encephalocele, what other abnormalities do Meckel–Gruber patients have?

Polycystic/dysplastic kidneys and polydactyly

Mnemonic:
Think of a little old man driving an *M-G* convertible in Florida. He's too short to see over the dash due to his small head. (The brain often atrophies with old age, but in this case, it's his whole head – especially since part of it is riding on his head rest – *occipital encephalocele*)

As with trisomy 13, too many fingers leads to too many holes in the kidneys! (*Polydactyly & polycystic kidney disease.*) He has a urinal in the passenger seat, in case he needs it for a long drive, but it's empty, because his kidneys are messed up!

Meckel–Gruber syndrome is lethal. Its inheritance pattern is _____?

Recessive
(Most very bad things are recessive – that's how these genes manage to survive to be passed on)

Small head, lissencephaly, and *vertical forehead wrinkles* go with what congenital syndrome?

Miller–Dieker
(lissencephaly means "smooth brain" – the gyral pattern is missing)

Mnemonic:
Think of a really dumb "MD" (no gyri), whose head is so shrunken that the skin on the forehead wrinkles vertically!

Agyria is an unusual condition in which the brain does not have a gyral pattern. Agyria is the "A" in HARD±E syndrome. What do the other letters stand for?

Hydrocephalus
Agyria
Retinal
Dysplasia
Encephalocele

What is the eponymic name for HARD±E syndrome?

Walker–Warburg syndrome

Agyria sounds like it means smooth brain, too. Is it different from lissencephaly?

No. They are the same

A short patient with a small head has eyelids that go *down* (ptosis) but nares that go *up*. She has MR and a cholesterol metabolism defect. What is the syndrome?

Smith–Lemli–Opitz

Cryptorchidism, hypospadias, syndactyly of toes #2 & 3, and a cholesterol metabolism defect = what syndrome?

Smith–Lemli–Opitz

Mnemonic:
SLO – MR is slow thinking, and the toe syndactyly gives them "sloth feet" – sloths are SLOw!

Renee Zellweger playing a character who is blind & retarded, and holding the little finger flexed, will help you to remember some important characteristics of what syndrome?

Zellweger (of course!)

(They also have "calcific stippling" of the epiphyses – little dots of calcium)

What metabolic problem do Zellweger patients have? (It leads to hepatomegaly)	Peroxisomal processing defects Mnemonic: Think of Renee Zellweger's character, applying H_2O_2 to her hair to make herself a blond, with her bent fingers!
Hepatomegaly with renal & GU issues + facial anomalies & metabolic problems = what (metabolic) syndrome?	Glutaric acidemia – Type II
Are glutaric acidemia patients acidotic?	**No**
Glutaric acidemia type II patients often have hepatomegaly and what other structural issues? (2 categories)	Renal/GU abnormalities Facial dysmorphologies
Low serum copper and skeletal & hair issues go with what X-linked syndrome?	**Menkes (kinky hair) syndrome** (aka Menkes "Steely" Hair Syndrome)
Syndromes that are named with big acronyms usually have what sort of inheritance?	Sporadic
Sexual precocity & light skin macules + bony growths = what syndrome?	**McCune–Albright Syndrome**
What does the "MURCS" syndrome stand for?	**MUllerian Renal aplasia Cervicothoracic- Somite dysplasia**
How can you remember that Edwards syndrome is trisomy 18?	Because Edwards begins with "E" & so does Eighteen
What are the three common trisomies?	**21 Down 18 Edwards 13 Patau's**
How can you remember the inheritance of Diamond–Blackfan syndrome?	Diamonds are the hardest substance – they're dominant! (Autosomal dominant)

How can you remember the inheritance of Holt–Oram syndrome?

"Holt!" sounds like "Halt!" –
A military police officer might say something like that – and they're dominant!

There are two syndromes, both having two-person eponymic names, that have *smooth* brains. What are they?

Miller–Dieker

&

Walker–Warburg

Miller–Dieker syndrome has the initials "MD." How can you use that to remember the disorder?

Think of a very dumb doctor (cortex smooth) with a small head & chin – the head is so small that there are vertical wrinkles on the forehead

(The wrinkles might even make an "M" to remind you of Miller–Dieker!)

What is a key difference between Miller–Dieker & Walker–Warburg?

- In Miller–Dieker the head is smaller
- In Walker–Warburg it is bigger (due to hydrocephalus)

Mnemonic: Mispronounce "Warburg" as "War-big" to remember that the head is big

Cornelia de Lange syndrome is also known as de Lange syndrome. What "hair findings" go with this syndrome?
(4)

1. **Low hairline**
2. **Hirsute**
3. **Synophrys (unibrow)**
4. **Long lashes**

Structural & growth abnormalities in de Lange syndrome usually go toward things being small. What are the abnormalities?
(4)

1. IUGR & postnatal growth retardation
2. Microcephaly
3. Micrognathia
4. Micromelia (small hands & feet or sometimes shortened limbs)

Cornelia de Lange patients sometimes have a serious structural problem. What is it?

Heart defects

Cornelia de Lange syndrome occurs sporadically. What are its main features?
  (4 groups)

1. **Smallness – IUGR, growth retardation, microcephaly, micrognathia, micromelia**
2. **Hair stuff – low hairline, single eye brow (goes across midline), long lashes, hirsute**
3. **Minor facial abnormalities**
4. **Heart defects**

What does the term "brachycephaly" mean?

A short, broad head

Is telecanthus different from hypertelorism?

No
(Both mean wide-set eyes)

Peutz–Jeghers is a mainly GI genetic disorder. What are its hallmarks?
  (3)

1. **Gut polyps/hamartomas**
2. **Freckling of lips, gums, genitalia**
3. **Increased risk of reproductive system cancers**

How is Peutz–Jeghers inherited?

AD –
Think of Frankenfurter from the Rocky Horror Picture Show – he had big prominent lips and was definitely a dominant character!

Before conducting genetic testing on a child, is it necessary to obtain consent?

Yes

If you are obtaining consent for genetic testing of a child, who should you obtain it from?

The parents – and the child should give his/her *assent* if ≥7 years old

What justifies conducting medical genetic testing?

"Timely" medical benefit
            Or
Psychosocial benefit

How is "timely" medical benefit defined?

Medical benefit prior to reaching adulthood

(Genetic testing of a child should be deferred until adulthood if there is no benefit to knowing the information earlier)

If parents wish to have a child tested for a genetic disorder, but the physician believes that the harm of testing is greater than the benefit, what is the physician supposed to do?

"Dissuade" the parents

If the benefits & harms of conducting a genetic test on an *adolescent* are unknown, whose wishes should the physician follow – the parents' or the adolescent's?

**The adolescent's
(Even if the two are in conflict)**

If a patient is less than 18 years old, and cannot give legal consent for genetic testing, should the risks, benefits, and explanation of the testing procedure still be given to him or her?

Yes

Can a patient less than 18 years old formally provide his or her agreement to participate in genetic testing?

Yes –
They can give "assent"

(agreeing, rather than giving permission or consent)

Are genetic disorders a cause of significant *morbidity* in the pediatric population?

**Yes
(40 % of admissions *to children's hospitals* involve genetic disorders)**

Are genetic disorders a significant cause of *mortality* in the pediatric population?

**Yes –
11 % of childhood deaths are related to genetic disorders**

Are all of the mitochondria in a single individual derived from an original, single, mitochondria in the egg?

No –
There is usually more than one mitochondria in the egg, & the mitochondrial DNA in each one is not necessarily the same

Why does it matter whether all of the mitochondria are the same or not?

Mitochondrial disorders may not affect all cells equally, because the cells "inherited" different mitochondrial lines

Some genetic disorders are called "gain-of-function" disorders. This makes no sense, because the patient has problems, not added benefits! What does a "gain-of-function" disorder mean? (3)

Three possibilities:

1. The protein is more effective than normal
2. Too much protein is being made
3. The protein is made in inappropriate situations

Name two of the more common "gain-of-function" genetic disorders.

1. Achondroplasia
2. Charcot–Marie–Tooth, type 1A (aka peroneal muscular atrophy)

One form of "loss of function" due to genetic errors is when a mutated recessive gene fails to produce an effective protein. This situation results in what two outcomes?

1. No phenotypic effect (no problem)
2. "Haploinsufficiency" (50 % of gene product is made, but that is not enough for normal function)

If a loss-of-function mutation produces a protein that *actually interferes with the function of the normal protein*, what is the special name for that?

Dominant negative effect

What does "haploinsufficiency" mean?

When production of a protein by just one gene is <u>not</u> enough for normal function

Microdeletion syndromes are sometimes also called _____?

Contiguous gene syndromes

What are "triplet repeat" disorders?

Genetic disorders that occur when too many copies of certain three base-pair sequences occur in the DNA

Name four famous triplet repeat diseases?

1. **<u>F</u>riedrich's <u>A</u>taxia**
2. **Fragile <u>X</u> (several types)**
3. **<u>My</u>otonic <u>D</u>ystrophy**
4. **<u>H</u>untington's <u>C</u>horea**

Mnemonic:
FAX, FAX, FAX for an MD to the HC (<u>H</u>ead <u>C</u>orters).
The three FAXs remind you that the disorders are triplet repeat syndromes
MD is for myotonic dystrophy
HC is for Huntington's chorea

How do triplet diseases work across generations?

The number of repeats tends to increase or "expand," worsening disease severity or making age of onset earlier

What is a modifier gene?

One that alters how an abnormal gene is expressed

Modifier genes can affect the expression (phenotype) of sickle cell disease. How?

Sometimes patients also inherit a gene for persistence of fetal hemoglobin in the circulation. Fetal Hgb does *not sickle*, so it makes the phenotype less severe

At what maternal age is genetic counseling routinely recommended?

≥35 years

At what *paternal* age is genetic counseling routinely recommended?

>50 years

Which ethnic groups should be screened for thalassemia to evaluate whether parents might be heterozygotes?

**Mediterranean
Arab
Indo-Pakistani**

Which ethnic groups are at special risk for Tay–Sachs & Canavan disorder (and should be screened for carrier status)?

Ashkenazi Jews
&
French-Canadians

Tay–Sachs is an autosomal recessive disorder with what hallmarks on physical exam?

Cherry red spot in retinal exam
Exaggerated startle response
Hypotonia

(3)

Sickle cell anemia affects a bigger segment of the world's population than thalassemia does. What ethnic groups should be screened for sickle cell status?

(Everywhere malaria is/was common)

**Mediterranean
Arab
Indo-Pakistani
Turkish
Southwest Asian
West African**

In approximately what percentage of cases is the gene responsible for a particular genetic condition known?

About 10 %
(Despite the human genome project, which gives us a good start)

Are most genetic disorders the result of a single "bad" gene?

No –
Outcome probably depends on certain genes more than others, but multiple gene and environment modify expression

In addition to the H&P and pedigree, what other steps are <u>required</u> for proper genetic counseling of a patient and family?
(3)

1. **Physical exam of family members not obviously affected**
2. **Support group info, along with <u>contact person</u>**
3. **Mechanism for updating when new info is discovered**

If you cannot make a specific diagnosis regarding a particular genetic disorder for a patient or a family, what should you do?

Explain the differential diagnosis

When a genetic disorder diagnosis is made, and you have thoroughly discussed it with the patient & family, what else are you expected to do?

Provide the information in writing

When a genetic disorder diagnosis is made, it is important to discuss the expected natural history of the disorder. If the specific prognosis is not clear, what must be discussed?

Best- & worse-case scenarios

In addition to providing all necessary contact information for support groups, you also need to provide patients with a genetic disorder with referrals to _____?

The relevant specialists

In addition to amniocentesis & chorionic villus sampling, DNA studies of fetuses can sometimes be performed noninvasively by sampling what?

Fetal blood in the maternal circulation

If a couple or an individual is at high risk for having a child with a bad genetic disease, what should you recommend in terms of whether to attempt further pregnancies?

The buzzword is "nondirective counseling"

(Meaning the health care provider must not bias the patients' choices in any way)

What are the three most common causes of an elevated alpha-fetoprotein (AFP) level?

1. Neural tube defect (anencephaly or open spina bifida)
2. Ventral wall defect
3. *Incorrect gestational age*!

What is the problem in Wilson's disease?

Too much copper in tissues

How is Wilson's disease inherited?

Autosomal recessive

An adolescent present with bizarre behavior and declining student performance. An unusual eye finding is noted on physical exam. What is the finding, and what is the diagnosis?

- **Kayser–Fleischer ring (golden-brown ring around the edge of cornea)**

- **Wilson's disease**

Wilson's disease mainly affects which parts of the body?

1. Liver
2. CNS

What unusual hematological finding goes with Wilson's disease?

Hemolytic anemia – *not immune*!

Which lab values are typically <u>high</u> in Wilson's disease?

1. Amount of copper in liver (from biopsy)
2. Urinary excretion of copper
3. Serum copper (sometimes)

Which important lab value is low in Wilson's disease?

Serum ceruloplasmin
(the molecule the body uses to transport copper)

How is Wilson's disease treated?
(Four levels of treatment)

1. Diet – decrease copper in food (nuts, chocolate, shellfish)
2. Zinc supplements – decrease gut absorption of copper
3. Chelation – Penicillamine or BAL
4. Transplant

A blond-haired, blue-eyed, pale child with mental retardation and a "musty odor" probably has what disorder?

Phenylketonuria

A deficiency of tetrahydrobiopterin produces what metabolic problem?

High phenylalanine –

So does lack of phenylalanine hydroxylase

Are both types of hyperphenylalanin-emia treated the same way?

Yes & no –

Both need restriction of phenylalanine –

Tetrahydrobiopterin deficiency also needs replacement (of tetrahydrobiopterin) & sometimes dopamine/serotonin supplementation

How is phenylketonuria inherited?

Autosomal recessive

How is phenylketonuria treated?

Dietary restriction of phenylalanine

If too much phenylalanine gets into the diet of a PKU patient, what problem will result?

Severe mental retardation

Are there special issues for pregnant phenylketonuric patients?

Yes – Phenylalanine levels must remain low (<10 mg/dL) to avoid fetal problems

If a pregnant PKU patient has phenylala-nine levels above 10 mg/dL, what are the likely consequences?

1. Spontaneous abortion
2. Mental retardation
3. Cardiac defects
4. Low birth weight

What are the main consequences of homocystinuria?

MR

&

Risk of thromboembolism

Homocystinuria patients look a lot like which other patient group?

Marfan's

What is the problem in homocystinuria?

Deficiency of cystathionine beta-synthase

How is homocystinuria inherited?	**Autosomal recessive** (When in doubt, guess autosomal recessive!)
Homocystinuria results in a buildup of which two molecules?	**Homocystine** **&** **Methionine**
How is homocystinuria treated?	1. Try pyridoxine – some patients respond to B_6 by itself 2. Give cysteine & folate 3. Restrict methionine in diet
How is Tay–Sachs inherited?	**Autosomal recessive**
Although other disorders also have this finding, what ophthalmological finding is a buzzword for Tay–Sachs?	**"Cherry red spot" on the retina**
What is the prognosis for children with Tay–Sachs?	**Death by 5 years**
A deficiency of the beta-hexosaminidase A enzyme causes what sort of problem?	**Lysosomal storage problems – Tay–Sachs disease**
A hypotonic, apathetic, infant presents to you. When you drop an instrument, you notice a pronounced _startle reflex_. What is the likely diagnosis?	**Tay–Sachs disease**
CNS degeneration begins by what age in Tay–Sachs children?	9 months
Tay–Sachs is most common in which ethnic group?	**Ashkenazi Jews**
What X-linked recessive disorder produces large but weak muscles early in childhood and can also affect the heart?	Duchenne muscular dystrophy
Dystrophin gene mutation produces what muscular disorder?	Duchenne muscular dystrophy

Which lab value is typically abnormal in Duchenne's muscular dystrophy?

Creatine kinase
(The muscle cells are having a problem, so CK goes up)

Which muscular dystrophy presents very much like Duchenne but symptoms begin later and progress more slowly?

Becker!!

What are the buzzwords for Duchenne muscular dystrophy on physical exam?
(2)

1. **Pseudohypertrophy of calves**
2. **Gower sign (using the arms to "walk up" the thighs when standing up)**

A short female presents with primary amenorrhea. What genetic disorder should be in the differential diagnosis?

Turner's syndrome

Structural ear abnormalities plus conductive hearing loss & facial asymmetry = what genetic syndrome?

Goldenhar

Retinitis pigmentosa + sensorineural hearing loss = what genetic syndrome?

Usher syndrome

Sensorineural hearing problems + white forelock of hair = what genetic syndrome?

Waardenburg

An infant with gram-negative sepsis that won't respond to antibiotics until a metabolic problem is corrected = which metabolic problem?

Galactosemia

A child develops "stork-like legs" & foot drop in adolescence. He has normal intelligence. Which *dominant* disorder is this?

Charcot–Marie–Tooth

Mnemonic:
Think of the legs being like "tooth" picks to help you remember the appearance

A *black liver, conjugated hyperbilirubinemia*, and an otherwise healthy patient = which recessive disorder?

Dubin–Johnson

What if a patient has a conjugated hyperbilirubinemia, but is otherwise well, and the liver is *not black*? Diagnosis?

Rotor syndrome

This autosomal dominant disorder causes behavior that will "dominate" a room – multiple tics, grunting, obscenities. Which disorder is it?

Gilles de la Tourette

Vomiting, jaundice, hepatomegaly, seizures, and *cataracts* go with what inborn error of metabolism?

Galactosemia

Telangiectasias of the GI tract, lungs, & brain – often with bleeding from the nose or the gut – indicates what genetic syndrome?

Osler–Weber–Rendu (aka hereditary hemorrhagic telangiectasia)

Mnemonic: Think of a man dancing the "rendu," an old-fashioned ballroom dance. He unfortunately develops a nosebleed, BRBPR, and starts coughing up blood while dancing. What a bad night!

Which syndrome has multiple *premalignant* intestinal polyps + supernumerary (extra) teeth?

Gardner syndrome

How is galactosemia inherited?

Autosomal recessive

Mnemonic:
The sugar problem "recedes" in their development, when it's corrected

How can you remember the inheritance of Osler–Weber–Rendu?

In the mnemonic, you are supposed to think of a *man* dancing – that is because men are supposed to lead, or dominate, in dance (autosomal dominant disorder)

What is an easy way to remember that Gardner syndrome is dominant?

Think of the crazed "gardener" who has genetically altered the plants so that their growth is out of control ("Dominant" plants with out-of-control growth to remind you of the malignant potential)

Childhood-onset polycystic kidney disease is a recessive disorder. What about adult PKD?

Dominant

A patient is presented with *weak muscles* and an *apathetic-looking face (apathetic facies)*. The child was born *breech*, with evidence of *arthrogryposis*. The condition seems to be *slowly worsening*. What is it?

Myotonic dystrophy
(autosomal dominant)

A patient presents with *seizures* and is found to be *hypocalcemic*. You note that the *4th and 5th metacarpals are shorter* than usual. What dominant disorder is this?

Albright hereditary osteodystrophy

(low calcium due to pseudohypoparathyroidism)

Mnemonic:
Albright was one of the founders of a German church. Dominant personalities found churches

Think of a church painted white with calcium, but the calcium is flaking off, to remember that their calcium level is low

What dominant disorder results in *oral ulcers*, and an increased risk of *C. perfringens* sepsis? (treatment is G-CSF)

Cyclic neutropenia (autosomal dominant)

A patient with *syndactyly of the 2nd and 3rd toes* presents with *elevated 7-dehydrocholesterol* on an exam! What is the disorder?

**SLO
Smith–Lemli–Opitz**

A 12-year-old patient presents with *ataxia. Posterior column function is abnormal*, and on exam you notice *high foot arches*. What is this child likely to die of?

Hypertrophic cardiomyopathy (Friedrich's ataxia)

Posterior columns = position & vibration info

Nodules over joints + hoarse voice = what diagnosis?

Farber syndrome

**Mnemonic:
The hoarse voice makes the patient seem shy or recessive – this disorder is (autosomal) recessive**

Neutropenia + malabsorption and steatorrhea = what diagnosis?	**Shwachman-Diamond**
A patient presents with fat malabsorption and onset of ataxia at 10 years old. A CBC is sent, and an unusual finding is reported for the RBCs. What is it?	**Acanthocytosis** (spiny projections on the RBCs) **(Diagnosis is abetalipoproteinemia)**
What recessive disorder causes deficiency of homogenetic oxidase and turns the urine black?	**Alkaptonuria**
Which two very unusual disorders are X-linked dominant?	Aicardi & Incontinentia pigmenti
A female patient is presented with an apparent hernia in the labial area. What diagnosis should be considered?	**Testicular feminization** (the hernia could be the testes)
A child who cannot feel pain has *episodes of hypertension*. What is the diagnosis?	**Riley–Day syndrome**
What is the underlying problem in Riley–Day syndrome?	CNS degeneration
Adrenoleukodystrophy patients may also have what acute life-threatening problem?	Adrenal insufficiency
Burning pain with *renal failure* is typical of galactosidase-A disorder?	Fabry disease
Self-mutilation & gout go with what X-linked recessive disorder?	**Lesch–Nyhan** (purine salvage pathway problem)
Missing sweat glands and *missing or abnormal teeth* suggest what X-linked diagnosis?	**Ectodermal dysplasia**

Chapter 4
General Inborn Errors of Metabolism Question and Answer Items

Inborn errors are usually inherited in what fashion?

Autosomal recessive
(second most common is X-linked)

New & trendy metabolic disorders are likely to be inherited in what fashion?

Mitochondrial

Can a patient inherit an X-linked disorder, yet have no prior family members affected?

Yes –
If Mom had the new mutation

Autosomal dominant inborn errors of metabolism are rare. These disorders usually affect what sort of body molecules?

Receptors or structural proteins
(e.g., familial hypercholesterolemia)

How can you identify a mitochondrial inheritance pattern?

• Passed via mother only
• Males & females all affected
(but penetrance may vary)

Should neurological syndromes due to errors of metabolism have focal features?

Generally, no

Acute encephalopathy with rapid progression, or occurring in very young infants, is often due to _____?

Inborn errors
(involving small molecules that can enter the brain)

What signs are usually present during pregnancy to tell you that the infant may have an inborn error?

None

C.M. Houser, *Pediatric Genetics and Inborn Errors of Metabolism: A Practically Painless Review*, DOI 10.1007/978-1-4939-0581-2_4, © Springer Science+Business Media New York 2014

Around the time of birth, how can you rapidly identify infants with inborn errors of metabolism likely to affect the CNS?

You can't
(The maternal circulation takes care of the metabolic processing error while in utero)

Small-molecule diseases that produce acute encephalopathy usually respond well to what management?

Hydration (IV)
(some dextrose to reverse catabolic states also helpful)

What general type of inborn error are you usually dealing with if there is a problem with muscle tissue?

Mitochondrial

If the reticuloendothelial system is affected by an inborn error of metabolism, what two disorder types are likely?

Lysosomal
    Or
Peroxisomal

Inborn errors of metabolism that affect organelles usually follow what type of course?

Gradual & progressive

Inborn errors of metabolism that affect organelles usually have what type of response to supportive (hydration) therapy?

Almost no response

Chronic encephalopathy + muscle weakness = what type of inborn disorder?

Mitochondrial

Intermittent ataxia is seen in which type of inborn errors?

Amino acid disorders

What is the only X-linked peroxisome disorder?

Adrenoleukodystrophy

(all others are autosomal recessive)

If you see problems in both the CNS & PNS, what two classes of inborn errors could be to blame?

Lysosomal
    Or
Peroxisomal

Lysosomal & peroxisomal inborn problems tend to cause defects in what three organ systems?

1. **Reticuloendothelial**
2. **CNS**
3. **PNS**

Early coronary artery disease suggests what inborn error?

Familial hypercholesterolemia

Early stroke suggests what inborn error?

Familial hypercholesterolemia

If you suspect an inborn error of metabolism, and discover that your patient is *hypoglycemic*, what does that tell you?

Inborn error is likely –
Doesn't tell you which one, though

What is a non-glucose-reducing substance?

Some other carbohydrate

If the patient's urine contains non-glucose-reducing substances, what categories of disorders should you consider?

Carbohydrate disease
       Or
Amino acid disease

Amino acid disorders usually have what effect on cognition?

Mental retardation

To diagnose an amino acid disorder, what two lab tests are most critical?

1. **Urine organic acids**
2. **Plasma amino acids**

Why do PKU patients have that "musty" odor?

Phenylacetic acid in the urine

Which enzyme is defective in PKU?

Phenylalanine hydroxylase (PAH)

If PAH does not function properly, what happens?

Phenylalanine builds up, because it cannot become tyrosine

At what age is the damage to the CNS from PKU irreversible?

8 *weeks*

In addition to the musty odor, PKU babies also often present with _____?
   (3 items)

1. Vomiting
2. Irritability
3. Eczema-like rash

Are most of the patients who test positive on the PKU screen actual PKU patients?

No –
Most are false positives

If the PKU screen is positive, what is the next test you should do?

Quantitate the tyrosine & phenylalanine levels

Is breastfeeding alright for PKU infants?

Yes

Is the ideal goal of therapy for PKU to eliminate phenylalanine in the diet?

No –
Some is needed for normal development

If a mother has untreated PKU, will it harm the fetus?

**Yes –
Heart defects
MR
IUGR
Microcephaly**

What is "hyperphenylalaninemia?"

High phenylalanine blood levels, without classic PKU

What are the clinical consequences of significant hyperphenylalaninemia?

Severe neurological effects including hypotonia & spasticity

An important subset of the hyperphenylalaninemia patients have what biochemical cause for their disorder?

Defects in synthesis or recycling of "biopterin"

Does hyperphenylalaninemia respond to the same intervention as PKU?

Not really –
It is not clear whether dietary changes are helpful, and they do cause nutritional risks

In addition to phenylalanine restriction, what other treatment is needed for patients with significant hyperphenylalaninemia?

Give biogenic amines

(That's dopa & 5-hydroxytryptophan)

The tyrosinemias refer to a group of disorders that have what in common?

High tyrosine levels

What is the most common type of tyrosinemia?

"Transient"
(common in preemies – resolves with maturation of the enzymes)

There are three types of genetic deficiency tyrosinemias. Type 3 is very rare. What do types 1 & 2 mainly affect?

Type 1: Hepatorenal
Type 2: Oculocutaneous

All of the tyrosinemias are treated with a low tyrosine diet. Type 1 is also treated with what?

NTBC

(A substance that blocks tyrosine metabolite – preventing buildup of toxins)

Mnemonic:.
Think of the NTBC acronym standing for Needs Tyrosine Blocking Compound!

What is ochronosis?

Pigment deposition in the ears & sclerae of *adult* alkaptonuria patients

(Pigment deposits in any connective tissue, actually)

When an alkaptonuria patient first voids a urine specimen, is it normal looking or dark?

Normal –
It turns dark as it stands (due to oxidation)

What is "infantile Parkinsonism?"

A tyrosine hydroxylase deficiency producing serious Parkinsonism (in infancy)

Some inborn errors involve the "branched-chain" amino acids. Which ones are those?

Valine
Isoleucine
Leucine

What lab test will diagnose a branched-chain amino acid defect?

Urine organic acid test

(plasma levels also helpful)

If a child has a normal phenylalanine level after dietary modifications, but the neurological disease continues to progress, what is the nature of the problem?

Hyperphenylalaninemia due to a "biopterin" problem

Why is biopterin biochemically important?

A form of it is required to make phenylalanine hydroxylase and the neurotransmitters serotonin & dopamine

What is the best known branched-chain amino acid disorder?

Maple syrup urine disease

Mnemonic:
That's how you remember that one of the first tests you send for these disorders is <u>urine</u> organic acids! It's in the name of this disorder. (Not very specific, though)

What helpful mnemonic involving a New England state helps you to remember the amino acids involved in maple syrup urine disease?

I = Isoleucine
Love = Leucine
Vermont = Valine
Maple syrup!

Is it only the urine that smells funny in maple syrup urine disease?

No –
Hair & skin also

What is the main goal of therapy for branched-chain amino acid defects?

Dietary control –
Restrict valine, isoleucine, & leucine in the diet

All patients with branched-chain amino acid defects should have a trial of what treatment?

Thiamine!
(One rare form responds well to thiamine)

Finding this abnormal amino acid in your patient's blood is *diagnostic* for maple syrup urine disease. What is the abnormal amino acid?

<u>**Allo**</u>**isoleucine**

Is there a milder version of branched-chain amino acid defect than maple syrup urine disease?

Yes –
Intermittent forms

How does intermittent branched-chain aminoaciduria present?

Episodes of:
ataxia,
lethargy, &
sometimes coma

Between episodes of intermittent branched-chain aminoaciduria, how do these patients present?

Normal

Do patients with intermittent branched-chain aminoaciduria usually have cognitive impairment?

No

If a patient has intermittent form branched-chain aminoaciduria, what determines when the episodes happen?

Stressors –
Often infection

There are two types of glutaric acidurias. What should you know about type 2?

They are going 2 die –
in the neonatal period
(100 %)

A macrocephalic infant develops normally until the age of 2½ years. Following a cold, he or she develops hypotonia & dystonia. What is the disorder?

Glutaric aciduria type 1

How can you diagnose glutaric aciduria type 1 before symptoms develop?

Check the urine
(increased glutaric acids in the urine)

Is glutaric aciduria type 1 treatable?

Yes

To be effective, when must glutaric aciduria type 1 treatment begin?

Before symptoms begin
(ideally in the neonatal period)

How is glutaric aciduria type 1 treated?

- Give L-carnitine
- Avoid lysine & tryptophan

Ocular lens dislocation is typically seen in what two disorders?

1. **Marfan's**
2. **Homocystinuria**

How are the lens findings different in Marfan's & homocystinuria?

Marfan's – usually upward
Homocystinuria – usually downward

Do homocysteine (homocystinuria) patients look like Marfan's patients?

Yes – but their joints are less flexible than usual

In addition to having limited joint flexibility, what else suggests homocystinuria, rather than Marfan's, as a diagnosis?

- Mental retardation
- Osteoporosis
- Lens dislocation downward

What is the classic cause of homocystinuria?

Cystathionine B-synthase deficiency

Does homocystinuria result from only one biochemical error?

No – there are at least six known causes

What cardiovascular issue do homocystinuria patients have?

Increased risk of thromboembolism (arterial & venous)

What is the first-line treatment for homocystinuria?

B12 – Large doses
(treats just one type, but it's worth a try!)

If your homocystinuria patient does not respond to B12 treatment, how should you treat him/her?

Give: L-cystine
Avoid: Methionine

Why is the medication "betaine" useful for patients with homocystinuria?

Allows homocysteine to convert to methionine
(alternative biochemical path)

What is hyperglycinemia?

High glycine levels (due to an inborn error)

Are hyperglycinemia patients acidotic or ketotic?

No

Why is it bad to have too much circulating glycine?

It concentrates in the CNS and causes intractable seizures

When do patients with maple syrup urine disease present?

**First week of life
(dead in 2–4 weeks without treatment)**

How do maple syrup urine disease infants present?

CNS symptoms –
- **Seizures & rigidity**
- **Loss of reflexes & respiratory irregularity**
- *Hypoglycemia*

What are the two main clinical consequences of hyperoxaluria?

Renal stones
&
Renal failure

How can hyperoxaluria be treated?

Liver
&
Kidney
Transplant

If the problem with hyperoxaluria is renal damage, then why isn't renal transplant enough to treat it?

Because the excess oxalate *is coming from the liver*!

What kind of renal stones do hyperoxaluria patients form?

Calcium oxalate

What is the difference between hyperoxaluria and "oxalosis?"

In oxalosis, oxalate deposits develop *outside the kidney*

If there is a problem with the urea cycle, why does that cause problems for the body, mainly?

Too much circulating ammonia

How does too much circulating ammonia harm the body?

It causes cerebral edema

How high does the ammonia level need to be to cause CNS symptoms?

About 100 μmol/L

On the boards, what is a good tipoff that you should consider a urea cycle disorder?

Septic looking infant with ABG showing *respiratory alkalosis* (*especially if it's a boy!*)

How is the elevated ammonia associated with urea cycle defects different from the elevated ammonia of patients with liver disease?

The ammonia is not different, <u>but</u> urea cycle patients should have normal (or near normal) LFTs

The urea cycle is a long pathway. How can you tell whether the defect is early or late in the cycle, clinically?

More severely affected individuals usually have earlier defects

Partial deficiencies for enzymes late in the cycle will sometimes show up after the neonatal period. When these deficiencies become evident, what is usually in the history?

A stressor (infection, injury, etc.)

Is the BUN high or low in urea cycle disorders?

LOW –
The defect is in producing urea, so blood *urea* nitrogen is low

In urea cycle defects, what is a citrulline level used for?

To differentiate early defects (low citrulline) from late ones (normal citrulline level)

How is a urinary orotic acid level useful in diagnosing urea cycle defects?

Elevated if OTC is the problem (Ornithine TransCarbamoylase)

In general, how are urea cycle defects treated?

Limit dietary nitrogen
Replace arginine
High calorie diet
Give sodium benzoate

(Restrict protein to limit dietary nitrogen)

How does sodium benzoate help patients with urea cycle defects?

It encourages alternate pathways for nitrogen processing

Which urea cycle defect is the only one that does <u>not</u> need arginine replacement?

Argininemia
(makes sense!)

Like the other inborn errors of metabolism, urea cycle defects are almost all inherited in what way?

Autosomal recessive

"Orotic" sounds like "ornithine."
A high urinary orotic acid level tells you _____?

That an OTC defect is the problem in the urea cycle
(ornithine transcarbamoylase)

An infant that smells of "sweaty feet" has what inborn error?

Isovaleric acidemia

What is the main problem isovaleric acidemia creates?

Acidosis

Will isovaleric acidemia present in the newborn period?

Not usually

Can isovaleric acidemia be treated in the long term?

Yes –
Prevent acidotic episodes by modifying diet

If infants or children survive their initial acidotic episode, what course will their isovaleric acidemia follow, without treatment?

Intermittent acidosis <u>with pancytopenia</u>

An infant presents with high ammonia, normal LFTs, and no ketones or acidosis. What diagnosis is likely?

Urea cycle defect

What causes propionic acidemia?

Deficiency of propionyl-CoA carboxylase
(PCC)

How does propionic acidemia present in the neonatal period?
(3)

1. High ammonia
2. Ketoacidosis
3. Bone marrow depression

When propionic acidemia presents in older infant & children, what unusual bone finding is often present?

Osteoporosis
(sometimes severe)

What is the prognosis for propionic acidemia?

Most die in early childhood

In general, how is propionic acidemia treated?

Avoid: Protein
Give: Carnitine
(increases excretion)

Alopecia + skin rash + encephalopathy = what disorder?

**Multiple
   Carboxylase
      Deficiency**

What two enzyme deficiencies lead to multiple carboxylase deficiency?

Biotinidase & holocarboxylase synthase

What is the general biochemical problem with multiple carboxylase deficiency?

Biotin is not incorporated into the carboxylases

How is multiple carboxylase deficiency treated?

**Give "free" biotin
(symptoms will reverse)**

Methylmalonic acidemias can present in two ways – what are they?

Ketoacidosis with hyperammonemia
Or
Ketotic hyper<u>glycinemia</u>

Methylmalonic acidemias are really a group of disorders. How do you make the diagnosis of methylmalonic acidemia?

Urine ketones

&

Methylmalonic acid (serum) level

In general, how are methylmalonic acidemias treated?

Restrict protein
Give carnitine

(& try B12 – some respond to it)

Glutaric acidemia (type 1) babies are macrocephalic at birth and have what findings on head CT at birth?

Frontal & cortical atrophy
(big head – atrophied brain)

Although the disorder is called glutaric acidemia, do the patients usually have a metabolic acidosis?

No

The symptoms that develop at the age of 2–3 years in glutaric acidemia patients results from what CNS changes?

Caudate & putamen (striatal) degeneration

Mevalonic acidemia patients have elevated blood & urine levels of mevalonic acid. How do these patients present?

Like a rheumatological disease –

Fever, arthralgia, rash, lymphadenopathy, and *subcutaneous edema*
(*odd finding – helps to differentiate it*)

Does mevalonic acidemia cause CNS problems?

Yes –
Developmental delay

What cellular process provides most of the energy for both cardiac and skeletal muscle?

Fatty acid oxidation

Where in the cell does fatty acid oxidation occur?

Mitochondria

The specific way fatty acids are oxidized is called _____?
(Chemical term)

β-oxidation
(produces energy)

What cofactor is necessary for the processing of fatty acids?

Carnitine

Fatty acid oxidation is also needed to generate what substitute energy substrate?

Ketones

Fatty acid oxidation disorders cause problems by disrupting four different steps. What are they?

1. Prevent β-oxidation
2. Prevent carnitine (cofactor) availability
3. Prevent fatty acids from entering mitochondria
4. Prevent ketone formation

What is the most common type of fatty acid oxidation defect?

MCAD
(**M**edium-**C**hain **A**cyl-coA **D**eficiency)

MCAD disorder children often present with what problems?

Muscle weakness
Cardiomyopathy
Arrhythmia
Destruction of muscle (exercise-induced rhabdo)

Which type of fatty acid oxidation defect is known as a particular cause of sudden infant death syndrome?

MCAD

At what age do MCAD patients usually present?

<2 years old

Does MCAD respond well to appropriate treatment?

Yes

What is the mainstay of treatment for MCAD deficiency?

Avoid fasting states

In addition to the heart, what other body organ is very affected by MCAD?

The liver

Elevated C_8, $C_{8:1}$, and $C_{10:1}$ esters indicate what kind of β-oxidation (fatty acid) defect?

MCAD
(**medium chain**)

In MCAD, do you expect to find high or low carnitine levels?

Low

In general, the longer the carbon chain an enzyme works on, the _____ the β-oxidation disease?

Worse!

In VLCAD (very long chain), how do most patients present?

Arrhythmias/sudden death Cardiomyopathy

In VLCAD, what esters allow you to make the diagnosis? (carbon molecules)

C_{14-18}

(carnitine is low again)

How do we treat acute episodes in β-oxidation disorders?

IV fluid & glucose

If you suspect a β-oxidation deficiency, and the patient also has *retinopathy*, what type of β-oxidation problem are you dealing with? (Pigment-based retinopathy)

LCHAD (Long-Chain Hydroxyl-coA Dehydrogenase)

Mothers of an affected fetus with which disorder are at increased risk for HELLP syndrome in pregnancy?

LCHAD

Cholestatic liver disease, in the setting of a β-oxidation disorder, means your patient has what type of β-oxidation problem?

LCHAD (long chain)

In addition to avoiding fasting, what other nutritionally based treatment is useful for long-chain and very-long-chain defects?

Give medium-chain triglycerides!

(Mediums will still be processed)

Elevated C_{16} and C_{18} esters are seen in which two β-oxidation defects?

Long chain (LCHAD)

&

Very long chain (VLCAD)

What is the underlying problem in the usually fatal glutaric acidemia type II?

Mitochondrial electron transport for both amino acid & fatty acid processing cannot happen

In carnitine uptake defect, or primary carnitine deficiency, what carnitine level do you expect to find in the blood?

Low

How is carnitine uptake defect or deficiency treated?

Give carnitine
(very good response)

How is L-carnitine given?

IV for acute episodes
Oral for maintenance

In addition to muscle weakness, carnitine deficiency can also present with what intermittent CNS problem?

Encephalopathy

CPT disorders refer to problems with what cofactor?

**Carnitine enzymes
(carnitine palmitoyl transferase)**

Carnitine enzyme disorders cannot affect the processing of which types of fatty acids?

Short

&

Medium chain

(They enter directly, without carnitine "escorting" them)

The overall general principle in managing fatty acid oxidation defects is to avoid _____?

Fasting

If serum ammonia needs to be removed acutely, how can that be done?

Dialysis

Glycogen is the storage form of _____?

Glucose

Glycogen metabolism defects lead to the development of what general class of disorders?

Glycogen storage diseases
(because the glycogen is not being removed)

There are two varieties of type 1 Glycogen storage diseases. Both have the same biochemical result. What is it?

Can't make glucose in the liver

(glucose-6-phosphate is not converted to glucose)

Which enzyme is defective/deficient in type 1 glycogen storage disease?	Glucose-6-phosphatase
How do von Gierke's (type 1) patients look?	Fat faces Big belly (large liver & kidneys) Skinny limbs Short stature
If you can't make glucose in your liver, you are at risk for what problem?	Fasting hypoglycemia
Von Gierke's (type 1) patients often have such profoundly low glucose that they present in early infancy with _____?	Seizures
In terms of lab tests, what unusual (fasting) profile is seen with type 1 glycogen storage disease?	↑ Lactate ↑ Lipids ↓ Glucose
How is the definitive diagnosis of type 1 glycogen storage disease made?	Genetic mutation analysis
How are the LFTs in von Gierke's disease?	Usually normal (despite the hepatomegaly)
Why are von Gierke's patients at increased risk for pancreatitis?	Elevated lipids (in particular, triglycerides)
Why would von Gierke's patients develop gout?	Chronically elevated uric acid levels (treat with allopurinol)
If type 1 glycogen storage disease patients have trouble with low fasting glucose levels, how can they be successfully managed during infancy? (von Gierke's)	Overnight glucose infusion (to the gut – not IV)
How are older von Gierke's patients managed overnight?	Corn starch before bedtime
Type 1b glycogen storage disease patients usually have a set of problems that the 1a patients don't. What problems are these?	1b has neutropenia & poor neutrophil function (recurrent bacterial problems)

In type III glycogen storage disease, what is the underlying biochemical problem?	Glycogen can't be debranched properly
Most patients with type III glycogen storage disease will have problems with what organ systems?	Both Liver & Muscle
Type III glycogen storage disease is most common in which two ethnic populations?	North African & Ashkenazi Jews
How is type III glycogen storage disease different in its presentation from type I?	1. No kidney involvement 2. Lactate & uric acid are normal (with glucose challenge, lactate will rise)
Type 0 (zero) glycogen storage disease is well named because the problem leads to _____?	<u>Less</u> glycogen than normal
What is the prognosis for type 0 disease?	Good
How is type 0 glycogen storage disease treated?	Frequent feedings to prevent hypoglycemia
"Hers disease" is type 6 glycogen storage disease. What is its prognosis & treatment?	Prognosis – Good No treatment (spontaneously resolves by puberty)
Type IV glycogen storage disease affects *many* organ systems. What is its usual course?	Death by 5 years due to cirrhosis
How do type IV glycogen storage disease patients usually present?	Liver cirrhosis Hepatomegaly Failure to thrive (by 18 months old)

Glycogen accumulating in the liver & kidney + proximal renal tubule dysfunction + rickets in a child less than a year old = what diagnosis?

Fanconi–Bickel

  aka

Type XI glycogen storage disease

(that's 11, for those weak on their Roman numerals!)

Consanguineous parents are often the source of this rare glycogen storage disease with proximal renal tubule dysfunction. What is it?

Fanconi–Bickel
(Type 11)

Although many glycogen storage diseases cause hepatomegaly, what is their usual effect on the LFTs?

None

Type XI glycogen storage disease causes what main long-term outcome? (aka Fanconi–Bickel)

Growth retardation/
Short stature

Is Fanconi–Bickel disease treatable? (aka type 11 glycogen storage disease)

No

Some glycogen storage diseases predominantly affect the liver, whereas others predominantly affect the muscles. Which ones mainly affect muscle?

2, 5, & 7

2 = Pompe's
5 = McArdle's
7 = Tarui's

Mnemonic:
2 + 5 = 7
In the Biblical story of Jacob, Egypt saves up grain for 7 years of famine. Think of them "storing" 7 years worth of carbs in the muscle to remember 2, 5, & 7

Pompe's disease (glycogen storage disease type II) is unusual because it affects which organ?

Often affects the <u>heart</u>

(*Mnemonic: Pompe – Pump*)

In all glycogen storage diseases, *except Pompe's*, the glycogen accumulates in which part of the cell?

The cytoplasm

In Pompe's disease (type II), where does the glycogen build up, and why?	• In the lysosomes • The enzyme deficiency is lysosomal!
There are three forms of Pompe's disease. What are they?	1. Infantile (worst) 2. Juvenile 3. Adult
Which of the three forms of Pompe's disease has cardiac involvement?	The infantile type (death before 1 year)
On EKG, what abnormality is especially common with Pompe's disease (infantile glycogen storage disease type 2)?	**Short PR interval**
Are the hearts of Pompe's babies enlarged?	Yes – And they are floppy due to weak muscles
If you do a muscle biopsy on a Pompe's patient, what do you expect to see?	Vacuoles full of glycogen
What lab test is likely to be high in type II glycogen storage disease that would not ordinarily be elevated with other, non-Pompe's, glycogen storage diseases?	CPK
How can type II (Pompe's disease) be definitively diagnosed?	• Test muscle cells or skin fibroblasts • Look for low acid glucosidase levels
What nighttime intervention sometimes improves the daytime symptoms of juvenile or adult Pompe's (type II) disease?	Ventilatory support
In addition to regular skeletal muscle problems, what more life-threatening problems do juvenile & adult-onset Pompe's patients have to endure? (2)	• Weak respiratory muscles • Swallowing problems
What is missing in Pompe's disease? (Type II glycogen storage disease)	Lysosomal acid α-1,4 glucosidase (for short, lysosomal acid glucosidase)

The lysosomal acid glucosidase that is missing in Pompe's (type II) disease also goes by another name. What is it?

Acid maltase

For infantile-onset Pompe's disease, what treatment can be attempted?

Enzyme replacement –
Good outcomes if started early in life

What diet modification is helpful for the juvenile- and adult-onset forms?

High-protein diet

McArdle's disease patients usually complain of what urinary symptom?

Red urine after exercise
(or at least dark)

What is the main danger of McArdle's disease?

Rhabdomyolysis damaging the kidney

What enzyme is abnormal (deficient) in McArdle's disease?

Muscle phosphorylase

If muscle phosphorylase is deficient, what chemical builds up with exercise?

**Ammonia –
Not lactate!**

Why does ammonia build up with exercise, rather than lactate, in McArdle's disease?
(Type 5 glycogen storage disease)

Glycogen/glucose conversion to lactate is impaired

(due to muscle phosphorylase deficiency)

(*For the interested – ammonia builds up due to abnormal ADP processing*)

What do glycogen storage disease type 5 mainly complain of?
(McArdle's disease)
(Three items)

1. Red urine after exercise
2. Exercise intolerance
3. Muscle cramps with exercise

How is type 5 glycogen storage disease diagnosed definitely?
(Two ways)

Gene analysis or enzyme assay on muscle tissue

What is helpful in the management of McArdle's disease?

1. Gradual exercise training
2. Avoid strenuous exercise
3. Glucose or fructose before exercise

If a patient has McArdle's disease, when is the disorder most likely to be troublesome?	Young adulthood
Type 7 glycogen storage disease (Tarui's disease) is very rare, but quite similar to McArdle's disease. How is it different?	1. Presents in childhood 2. Has hemolysis 3. Carb loading makes the exercise intolerance significantly worse
How is Tarui's disease (type 7) treated?	Avoid strenuous exercise
Glucose consumption before exercise is helpful with which glycogen storage disease?	Type 5 (McArdle's)
Why would glucose consumption before exercise actually harm performance in type 7 disease?	Ample glucose inhibits lipolysis – That's the energy source the muscle needs (because it can't process glucose)
Oddly enough, galactosemia patients are at increased risk of what infectious disease?	*E. coli* **sepsis** (*often precedes the galactosemia diagnosis!*)
When treating a galactosemia patient for sepsis, what is unusual about the response to treatment?	**Often won't respond until galactosemia is corrected**
What is the overall problem in galactosemia?	**Galactose can't be metabolized, so it builds up**
What two sugars combine to form lactose?	Glucose & galactose
What enzyme is deficient in galactosemia?	<u>**Galactose-1-phosphate uridyl transferase**</u>
Where does galactose-1-phosphate build up in galactosemia? (Which organs)	**Brain** **Liver** **Kidney** Mnemonic: Think of a BL<u>K</u> sandwich – topped off with a nice milkshake full of galactose to remind you of where the galactose builds up

When should an infant be tested for galactosemia?	**Newborn –** **Should be a standard screen**
How is the screening for galactosemia done?	**Fluorescent spot test for GALT activity**
Galactosemia has the usual findings on physical exam & labs (low glucose, big liver, etc.). What unusual findings will galactosemia patients have?	**Cataracts** **&** **Vitreous hemorrhage**
What is required to definitively diagnose galactosemia?	**Deficient enzyme** **GALT +** **Galactose-1-phosphate excess**
Although galactosemia patients often have some long-term problems, the liver, kidney, and ocular effects of galactosemia can be corrected. How?	Eliminate galactose from the diet
Will AST & LDH be elevated in type II glycogen storage disease (Pompe's disease)	Often, yes (Especially in the infantile form – look for ↑ CPK, also)
A hereditary galactose disorder that produces cataracts only is named _____?	Galactokinase Deficiency (Eliminate dietary galactose)
If a patient presents with cataracts, cirrhosis, HSM, mental retardation, & vomiting, you would think of possible galactosemia. If the patient was also *hypotonic* and had *nerve deafness*, what is the correct diagnosis?	UDP Gal-4 epimerase deficiency
How is UDP Gal 4-epimerase deficiency treated?	Take galactose out of the diet
A galactosemia presentation + what two features point you toward the UDP Gal 4-epimerase diagnosis?	Nerve deafness & Hypotonia

Is UDP Gal 4-epimerase deficiency always a bad diagnosis?

No –
There are two forms –
One is benign & requires no treatment

Hereditary fructose intolerance (aka aldolase B) presents much like galactosemia, but without ocular findings. In what other way is its presentation different?

Presents later –
Usually upon exposure to juice or sweetened cereal

How is aldolase B deficiency definitively diagnosed?

Assay for the enzyme's activity in the liver/genetic testing

If a patient is fructose intolerant, and fructose is removed from the diet, what will happen to the diseases' progress?

Damage reverses

If a patient is fructose intolerant, what sugars, *in addition to fructose*, must be avoided?

Sucrose

&

Sorbitol

If a patient presents with an acute episode of jaundice, HSM, lethargy, & vomiting, what should you check for in the urine?

Reducing substances (fructose, in particular)

If a patient has fructose in the urine, but no symptoms, what should you do?

Nothing –
It's benign fructosuria

How is Menkes disease inherited?

X-linked

Menkes disease patients, after the first week of life, will have what type of copper levels in their serum (and ceruloplasmin levels, as well)?

Low

Can Menkes disease be treated?

Partly –
Give copper histidinase injections before neural symptoms begin

Is the hair of Menkes patients really kinky?

Only on microscopic inspection

(It is noticeably brittle, though)

What is the other name sometimes given to Menkes kinky hair disease?

Menkes "steely" hair disease

What is the clinical presentation of Menkes disease?
  (4 components)

- **Hypoglycemic boy**
- **Fat face with "sagging jowls & lips"**
- **Temperature instability**
- **Sparse, light-colored, brittle hair (including eyebrows)**

At what age does the neurological part of Menkes usually begin?

2–3 months
(seizures,
loss of milestones)

What is the basic problem in Smith–Lemli–Opitz syndrome?

Defect in cholesterol synthesis

Smith–Lemli–Opitz syndrome reliably causes mental retardation and affects many systems. Why?

Cholesterol is critical to development

Smith–Lemli–Opitz syndrome patients can often be recognized by their abnormalities in what three areas of the body?

Extremities
Genitalia
Face

(Facial: micrognathia, wide eyes, wide nose tip, wide lids)

What do peroxisomes do?

Digest things using H_2O_2
(& other substances)

What are the three main molecules that peroxisomes digest?

1. Long-chain fatty acids
2. Amino acids
3. Uric acid

Generally speaking, what is wrong in Zellweger syndrome?

Multiple peroxisome functions are defective

What radiological finding is a hallmark of Zellweger syndrome?

"Calcific stippling" (dots) on the patella & long-bone epiphyses

X-linked adrenoleukodystrophy results from a defect in what organelle?	Peroxisome (a single peroxisome function is affected)
About 1/3 of patients with X-linked adrenoleukodystrophy have the childhood form. What happens in that disorder?	Central demyelination (between ages 3 & 10 years)
How does X-linked adrenoleukodystrophy involve the adrenals?	Most patients have adrenal insufficiency
Which version of X-linked adrenoleukodystrophy is most severe?	The childhood form – Fatal –
What lab test is helpful in making the X-linked adrenoleukodystrophy diagnosis?	Elevated very-long-chain fatty acids in serum (especially $C_{26:0}$)
What two syndromes have the following triad of problems: ptosis, ophthalmoplegia, ragged-red fiber myopathy?	1. Kearns–Sayre 2. Chronic progressive external ophthalmoplegia (CPEO) syndrome
If CPEO involves other organ systems, what is it called?	CPEO-plus syndrome
Kearns–Sayre, CPEO, and CPEO-plus, all result from problems with what cellular organelle?	Mitochondria
Are Kearns–Sayre, CPEO, and CPEO-plus usually inherited?	No – They are usually new mutations during development
At what age do CPEO and CPEO-plus usually become symptomatic?	Adolescence or adulthood (& worsen with age, too)
At what age does Kearns–Sayre present?	Can be as early as infancy
Of the three disorders, CPEO, CPEO-plus, and Kearns–Sayre, which one is most severe?	Kearns–Sayre

In addition to the triad of ptosis, ophthalmoplegia, & ragged-red fiber myopathy, what other problems often develop with Kearns–Sayre syndrome? (4)

Cardiomyopathy
Ataxia
Deafness
DM

Mnemonic:
If you develop all these problems, you will need a "CADDy" on the golf course. Think of a famous golfer named "Kearns Sayre" riding around with his CADDy

In MERRF, what is the usual pattern for myoclonic jerking?

The occur at rest & increase with movement

What is the triad of MERRF?

1. Epilepsy/myoclonic jerks
2. Ragged-red fiber disease
3. Cerebellar ataxia

When are patients with MERRF usually diagnosed?

Late childhood or later

Diabetes & stroke in a young person should make you consider what class of disorders?

Mitochondrial

(aka "oxidative phosphorylation diseases")

What does MELAS in "MELAS syndrome" stand for?

Mitochondrial Encephalomyopathy
Lactic Acidosis
Stroke-like episodes

In MELAS syndrome, what usually presents first – the ataxia or the stroke?

Ataxia

In addition to ataxia, stroke, and muscle problems, what other problem may develop for MELAS patients?

Cardiomyopathy

The famous "Friedrich's ataxia" is caused by a problem in which cellular organelle?

Mitochondria

(But the problem is in the cell's genome – the gene product is needed by mitochondria for oxidative phosphorylation)

(Transmission is autosomal recessive)

Friedrich's ataxia patients usually have what problems?

1. **Cardiomyopathy**
2. **Ataxia & ↓ DTRs**
3. **DM**

In addition to cardiomyopathy, ataxia, and diabetes, Friedrich's patients also have problems with two other aspects of the nervous system. What are they?

1. Corticospinal tract dysfunction
2. Vibration & proprioception sensations

In mucopolysaccharidoses (MPS), will the diagnosis usually be evident at birth?

No –
It develops as the (extra) stored material develops

Hurler syndrome is MPS type 1. What determines its prognosis?

The cardiac disease

(Cardiomyopathy & coronary artery disease)

Hurler syndrome kids have large head circumferences and are at risk for what deadly traumatic problem?

Atlantoaxial subluxation

Mnemonic:
Think of them "hurling" their heads!!

What sensory problems often affect Hurler syndrome kids?

Corneal clouding

&

Deafness

Mnemonic:
That's how you keep Hunter's & Hurler's syndromes straight – You can't "hunt" with bad vision & hearing

How does the face look in classic Hurler syndrome?

Coarse –
with large tongue & midface hypoplasia

How much variation is there in the severity of Hurler syndrome?

Huge –
Some don't present until adulthood

Sleep apnea problems in a kid with a big head & large tongue should make you consider which genetic disorder?

Hurler syndrome

All Hurler syndrome patients
eventually develop what problem?

Vertebral bone problems

&

Skeletal growth retardation

(The vertebral problems are
degeneration & spondylolisthesis)

What is special about MPS I S, also
known as Scheie syndrome (a variant
of Hurler syndrome)?

It is one of the three MPS disorders
with *normal intelligence*

Which other MPS disorders have
patients with normal intelligence?
(2)

Morquio syndrome
(MPS type 4)

&

Maroteaux–Lamy
(MPS type 6)

**MPS type 1 (Hurler syndrome) can
sometimes be treated, if treatment is
instituted early (<18 months). How
can Hurler's be treated?**

Bone marrow transplant

**When treatment for Hurler syn-
drome is successful, most of the
associated problems are avoided.
Which ones are not?**

The bony problems

Will bone marrow transplant work for
other types of MPS?

No –
Just type 1 (Hurler's)

Hunter syndrome is MPS II. In its
severe form, it is similar to MPS I. How
can you tell them apart?

- Hunter's live longer (mid-teens)
- *No corneal clouding* (Remember
  that hunters need good eyes!)

**What is very important about the
inheritance of Hunter's syndrome
(MPS type II)?**

It is the <u>only X-linked</u> MPS

**There is a pathognomonic skin rash
that sometimes affects Hunter (type
II) patients. What is it?**

A scapular & extensor surface rash

Mnemonic:
It's the area involved in holding your
rifle, if you're a hunter!

Is atlantoaxial instability a problem for Hunter syndrome patients?	No – That's Hurler's Mnemonic: Think of them "hurling" their heads!
Is sleep apnea a problem for Hunter syndrome (type 2) patients?	Yes – (but it usually presents later than in Hurler's patients)
Do Hunter's patients have bone or joint problems?	Yes
Which MPS is inherited in an X-linked fashion? (Give both names)	Type II Hunter syndrome
"Odontoid dysplasia" is an unusual problem. Which MPS causes it? (Give both names)	Type 4 Morquio syndrome
While odontoid dysplasia refers to a problem in the c-spine, these patients often also have problems with a nearby area with similarly named structures. What is it?	**The teeth** (especially dental decay)
What is the overall consequence of type 4, Morquio syndrome, MPS?	Bone problems (including bone-like structures, such as teeth)
What is the worst problem Morquio patients have to deal with, and why is it so bad?	• **Odontoid dysplasia** • **Produces cervical myelopathy**
Are Morquio patients dysmorphic? (In the face)	No
What two important aspects of type 4 MPS patients (Morquio syndrome) are completely normal?	**IQ** & **Facial features**
What happens to Morquio syndrome patients in terms of stature?	**"Short-trunk" dwarfism** (only about 3½ feet tall)

What eye finding goes along with Morquio syndrome?

"Fine corneal deposits"

What is the underlying problem in MPS type 4 (Morquio)?

Deficiency of glucose-6-sulfatase

Why is it a problem if you don't have enough glucose-6-sulfatase? (Biochemically speaking)

Keratan sulfate can't be degraded (this causes bone problems)

Sanfilippo syndrome is a type of MPS. Which type is it?

3

What is the underlying biochemical problem in type 3 MPS? (Sanfilippo syndrome)

Inability to break down *heparan* sulfate

What is unique about Sanfilippo syndrome – compared to the other MPS?

Very big effect on the CNS (compared to other body systems)

Since type III MPS affects the CNS so profoundly, what behavioral changes are expected with this syndrome?

Hyperactivity

&

Aggression

What is the "classic" pattern of CNS deterioration in Sanfilippo syndrome?

Three phases –
1. Developmental delay
2. Hyperactivity & aggression
3. Swallowing dysfunction & vegetative state

If a vignette describes what sounds like a Hurler's syndrome patient, but it specifically mentioned *hyperplastic gums*, what disorder are they looking for?

I-cell deficiency

Technically, I-cell deficiency is a mucolipidosis. What is the underlying problem that causes this disorder?

Lysosomal enzymes are missing a critical segment, so they can't find the lysosome!

In addition to hyperplastic gums, what other findings point toward I-cell deficiency (mucolipidosis type 2)?

Small head circumference

&

Frequent formation of new periosteal bone

Pseudo-Hurler polydystrophy is actually a mucolipidosis, but it closely resembles Hurler's. What are its main features?

(4)

1. Bad joint stiffness
2. Fairly normal life-span
3. Mild cognitive issues
4. No mucopolysaccharides in the urine

A patient who seems to have Hurler's but who also has a cherry-red spot on the retina probably has what disorder?

Cherry red spot myoclonus syndrome

(Mucolipidosis type 1)

Sialic acid genetic diseases are mainly seen in people from what small ethnic group?

Finnish

There are two main sialic acid diseases. What is the name for the mild disorder?

Salla disease

**Mnemonic:
Sounds almost like "sialic!" Think of it as "Siallic disease"**

What are the main complaints for patients with Salla disease?

Learning problems

What is the underlying problem in Salla disease?

A defect in the sialic acid transporter

Infantile sialic acid storage disease is a very serious form of sialic acid disease. What are its three main presentations?

1. Failure to thrive
2. Hydrops fetalis
3. Severe infections

In general, glycoproteinoses tend to affect which body system most commonly?

Immune system

What does sphingolipidosis have to do with lysosomes?

These disorders develop when lysosomal enzymes can't break down "sphingolipids"

What is the biochemical name for the stuff that builds up in all sphingolipidoses?

Ceramide

In each sphingolipidosis, two molecules accumulate: ceramide and one other. What are the two options for the other molecule?

**Oligosaccharide
Or
Phosphorylcholine**

What determines whether oligosaccharide or phosphorylcholine are produced, along with ceramide, in a sphingolipidosis?

If a glycosphingolipid was processed → oligosaccharide

Sphingomyelin → phosphorylcholine

Mnemonic:
The "phs" stay together!

Gaucher's disease is a type of sphingolipidosis. How many varieties of Gaucher's disease are there?

Four

What are the names of the sphingolipidoses you should know fairly well?

1. Gaucher's (four types)
2. Niemann–Pick (three types)
3. Fabry disease
4. Tay–Sachs

Which sphingolipidosis is X-linked?

Fabry

Which sphingolipidosis affects *only* the CNS?

Tay–Sachs

Which sphingolipidosis affects many body systems, including the PNS, but spares the CNS?

Fabry disease

Which type of Gaucher's disease presents earliest & most severely?

4 –
Neonatal presentation & death

What is unusual about the skin exam of a newborn with type 4 Gaucher's?

Thick & shiny "collodion" skin

(looks like parchment wrapped around the body)

What type of Gaucher's disease is most common?

Type 1

Does Gaucher's disease type 1 affect the CNS?

No

Gaucher's disease is most common in what ethnic group?

Ashkenazi (East European) Jews

What is the most common presentation of Gaucher's disease type 1?

Incidental splenomegaly on exam

Which sphingolipid-processing enzyme is missing in Gaucher's disease type 1?	**Glucocerebrosidase**
All of the types of Gaucher's disease involve problems with which enzyme?	**Glucocerebrosidase (but different tissues are affected in the different types)**
When diagnosing Gaucher's disease, the lab assays for a slightly different enzyme than the one responsible for the disorder. Which enzyme is it?	β-**glucosidase**
Samples of what cells will be needed to test for Gaucher's disease? (For enzyme testing)	**Leukocytes** Or **Skin fibroblasts**
If a type 1 Gaucher's patient has a bleeding crisis, what is usually required?	**Splenectomy (the platelets are being sequestered in the spleen)**
How is Gaucher's disease usually treated (type 1)?	**Enzyme infusion every other week controls disease progression**
What is a Gaucher's "bone crisis?"	When infiltrating cells cause bone pain (usually requires narcotics)
Why is enzyme therapy not much used for Gaucher's types 2, 3, & 4?	**It only treats the hematologic & bone problems**
What other sphingolipidosis presents very much like Gaucher's disease, type 1?	**Niemann–Pick type B** Mnemonic: They will <u>B</u> basically normal!
What is the histological buzzword for Niemann–Pick disorders in general?	**"Foamy" histiocytes**
Type B Niemann–Pick also has what poetically named cell on histology?	**"Sea blue" histiocytes** Mnemonic: <u>B</u>lue is for type <u>B</u>!!

Which three sphingolipidoses leave the CNS alone?	**Gaucher's type 1** **Niemann–Pick type B** **Fabry disease**
Which of the three sphingolipidoses that spare the CNS cause mainly hepatosplenomegaly?	Gaucher's disease, type 1 Niemann–Pick, type B
How many types of Niemann–Pick are there (in pediatrics)?	Three (Types A, B, & C)
Why is Niemann–Pick type B so mild?	The missing enzyme is present in lower amounts than usual, but still present
Niemann–Pick disorders are most common in what ethnic group?	**Ashkenazi Jews**
How does Niemann–Pick type A present?	**Vomiting, diarrhea, & failure to thrive early in infancy** **Then,** **hypotonia & loss of movement**
How common is Niemann–Pick type A?	Very rare Mnemonic: Thank heavens, because type <u>A</u> is <u>A</u>wful!
In a general way, how is Niemann–Pick type C different from the underlying pathophysiology of types A & B?	**Type C has to do with accumulation of cholesterol in the lysosome –** **It is not a true lysosomal enzyme defect at all!**
Which type of Niemann–Pick is most common?	**Type C**
How do Niemann–Pick, type C, kids present? (3)	Hepatosplenomegaly (90 %) Impaired cognition/fine motor skills Ataxia

What unusual neurological findings do Niemann–Pick type C patients often have?

(3)

1. Narcolepsy ("attacks" of sleep during otherwise alert periods)
2. Cataplexy (sudden loss of motor movement after scares, etc.)
3. Supranuclear gaze palsy (can't look up)

What is the gold standard for diagnosing Niemann–Pick type C?

Fibroblast culture shows (unesterified esters) cholesterol building up in lysosomes

What is the prognosis for Niemann–Pick type C?

Death in teens

If a Niemann–Pick type C patient has gaze palsy, what will you obtain if you test for "doll's eyes" movements?

Doll's eyes are intact (because it is a lower, non-voluntary function)

Comparing Gaucher's types 2 & 3, which one starts earlier?

Type 2 (But remember that Type 4 is <u>earliest</u> – neonatal)

What is the classic histology finding for Gaucher's disease – in general?

Large, basophilic histiocytes with "_crinkled tissue paper_" cytoplasm

Which two organ systems are mainly involved in type 2 Gaucher's?

**Liver –
big HSM (but LFTs are relatively normal)
Neural –
swallowing, eyes, posturing**

How early will type 2 Gaucher's patients begin to have problems?

Around 3 months

How is type 2 Gaucher's treated?

**It's not –
Death before age 2 is typical**

How many types of Tay–Sachs are there?

**Two –
Infantile**

&

Juvenile/adult

What is the classic physical exam finding for Tay–Sachs? (Although it does occur in other disorders)

"Cherry-red" spot on the macula

What unusual responses to auditory stimuli are seen in Tay–Sachs infants? (2)

1. Enhanced startle
2. Seizures

A normal Moro startle reflex decreases when the stimulus is repetitive. What pattern of response is seen in Tay–Sachs infants?

No decrease in startle with repetition

What is the prognosis for the infantile form of Tay–Sachs?

Death in early childhood

What is the prognosis for the juvenile/adult-onset Tay–Sachs?

Normal life-span,
But usually unable to ambulate in later life

What unusual pattern of muscle weakness do infantile Tay–Sachs patients present with?

Axial *hypotonia*,
But extremity hypertonia & hyperreflexia

When Tay–Sachs occurs in the juvenile form, when does it usually present?

School age

What are the main problems experienced by patients with juvenile Tay–Sachs?

1. Intention tremor
2. Dysarthria
3. Proximal muscle weakness
4. Mood disorders

The inability to break down heparan sulfate leads to which MPS?

Type 3
Sanfilippo

Which MPS disorder classically follows a triphasic pattern of symptoms?

Sanfilippo
1. Delay & diarrhea
2. Hyperactivity & aggression
3. Swallowing problems & vegetative state

Mnemonic:
Type 3 has three phases.

The underlying problem in the MPS Sanfilippo syndrome is?

Inability to break down heparan sulfate

Gaucher's disease type 3 actually has two types, 3a & 3b. How does 3a affect patients?

CNS dysfunction,
Including seizures, spasticity, &
oculomotor problems

Gaucher's disease type 3b initially presents mildly, like type 1. How is its course different?

Liver impairment proceeds
rapidly → ascites, portal HTN,
and coagulopathy

Is bone marrow transplant a helpful therapy for Gaucher's type 3b?

For the liver & hematologic prob-
lems, yes

(generally won't affect CNS problems)

Defective breakdown of keratan sulfate leads to what MPS disorder?

Morquio syndrome
(Type 4)

Mnemonic:
The "k" is keratan sounds like the "qu" in Morquio!

Although Fabry disease is an X-linked sphingolipidosis, what symptoms are sometimes seen in female carriers?

Pain crisis

How do Fabry patients present?

Episodes of hand & foot pain
beginning at puberty

What is the typical trigger for pain crises in Fabry patients?

Heat exposure
          Or
Heat exposure +
physical exertion

What do the pain crises of Fabry patients seem to be due to?

Peripheral neuropathy

If a Fabry patient is having difficulty with peripheral neuropathy pain, what regimen may control the pain?

Carbamazepine,
Gabapentin, etc.

(antiseizure meds often effective for peripheral neuropathy pain syndromes)

In addition to painful peripheral neuropathy, what other problems do Fabry patients have?

1. **Vessel problems – skin rash due to ectatic vessels, renal failure, coronary artery disease, stroke**
2. **Autonomic dysregulation**

The classic vignette for a Fabry patient is an adolescent male with hand & foot pain after _____?

Exercising in heat

An adolescent male presents in severe pain and is *not* sweating despite a hot environment. What is the disorder?

Fabry

(Lack of sweating is one part of their autonomic dysfunction)

"Maltese crosses" in the urine go with which sphingolipidosis?

Fabry

(The crosses are lipid globules in the urine, by the way)

Which enzyme deficiency causes the problems in Fabry disease?

α-galactosidase

Does Fabry disease affect the CNS?

No

Which of the sphingolipidoses do not affect the CNS?

1. Fabry
2. Gaucher's type 1
3. Niemann–Pick type B

How is the neurological involvement of Gaucher's disease type 3 different from that of type 2?

Type 3 begins later (school age)

&

Progresses more slowly

All forms of Gaucher's disease involve some degree of impaired function in which two body systems?

1. **Liver/spleen (with HSM)**
2. **Bone (due to infiltration)**

There are five common mutations that produce Gaucher's disease. How useful are these mutations for detecting Gaucher's in the Ashkenazi population?

Very useful –
97% of Gaucher's patients/carriers will be detected

How useful are the five common Gaucher's mutations when screening for the disease in the general population?	Useful – 75 % of Gaucher's will be detected
There are two general categories of porphyria, hepatic & erythropoietic. Which type leads to abdominal pain, neurological, and psychiatric disturbance?	**The hepatic**
Acute intermittent porphyria is the disorder King George of England may have had. It is a hepatic por-phyria. How is it inherited? (*The Madness of King George* depicted it on film!*)	**Autosomal dominant**
What does the board like to test, when they have a question on acute intermittent porphyria?	**The drugs that may precipitate an attack**
What is the typical presentation of acute intermittent porphyria?	**Episodes of abdominal pain, peripheral neuropathy seizures, & psychiatric changes**
What type of diet can induce a porphyria episode?	**Low calorie (Glucose infusions can be helpful in treating)**
What lifestyle/recreational choices make an attack of acute intermittent porphyria more likely?	**Recreational drugs & Alcohol**
Which prescription medications are most often implicated in attacks of acute intermittent porphyria? **(4)**	1. **Endogenous & exogenous gonadal steroids** 2. **Griseofulvin** 3. **Sulfonamides** 4. **Antiseizure meds, in general**
Although acute intermittent porphyria patients have abdominal pain, what will you find on abdominal exam?	No reliable tenderness (The abdominal pain is neurological)

If a porphyria patient has a seizure, what should you use to treat it?	**Clonazepam** **Or** **Bromides**
Weakness, due to peripheral neuropathy during an acute intermittent porphyria episode, follows what course?	It will return to normal but can take years to do so (or sometimes only days)
What is the best treatment for an acute attack of porphyria?	**Infusions of heme for several days at the start of the attack**
What lab test <u>rules out</u> acute intermittent porphyria, if it is normal?	**Porphobilinogen**
What is the most common porphyria?	**The werewolf one – Porphyria <u>cutanea</u> tarda**
How can you remember that porphyria cutanea tarda is the werewolf one, in terms of symptoms?	**Cutanea = skin** **Tarda = stays out late! (like tardy)**
What are the symptoms of porphyria cutanea tarda?	1. **Photosensitivity (breaks out in blisters)** 2. **Hyperpigmentation** 3. **Hypertrichosis (hairy)**
How is porphyria cutanea tarda treated?	**Bizarrely, phlebotomy** (Typically, removal of about 5 units of blood, 1 unit at a time, will cure or control it)
Which medications are helpful in the treatment of porphyria cutanea tarda?	**Chloroquines** (very small doses)
Why are chloroquines helpful in treating porphyria?	**They increase the excretion of the porphyrins that are building up**
Why is phlebotomy useful in porphyria cutanea tarda?	**It reduces the overall iron load**
Porphyrias, in general, are the result of what problem?	**A defect in the pathway generating hemoglobin → too many porphyrins**

X-linked sideroblastic anemia has what characteristic finding on bone marrow histology?	Sideroblasts
What causes the problem in X-linked sideroblastic anemia?	An RBC enzyme is deficient, decreasing effective erythropoiesis
How does X-linked sideroblastic anemia present?	**Infant male develops "refractory" microcytic anemia**
How then can you treat X-linked sideroblastic anemia? **(2)**	1. **B_6 works for some patients** 2. **Transfusions, then chelate to deal with complications of multiple transfusions**
Redness, burning, itching, & swelling of the skin within minutes of sun exposure indicate which porphyria diagnosis?	**Erythropoietic protoporphyria (EPP)**
Are any other skin findings common in EPP?	NO – Not even blisters!
What is the most common porphyria?	**Porphyria cutanea tarda** **Mnemonic:** **It's <u>common</u> to be <u>late</u>/tardy.**
What general type of porphyria is porphyria cutanea tarda – hepatic or erythropoietic?	Hepatic
What is the most common *erythropoietic* porphyria? (& second most common porphyria overall)	EPP
Which two erythropoietic porphyria are you supposed to know?	EPP & X-linked sideroblastic anemia
What diet modification is helpful for patients with EPP, and why?	• **β-carotene supplement** • **Improved sunlight tolerance**

What are the basic features of adenylate deaminase deficiency?

Muscle weakness

&

Cramping after vigorous exercise

To what general category of disorder does adenylate deaminase belong?

Purine disorders

How common is adenylate deaminase deficiency?

Very common (1–2 % of population), but often asymptomatic

What is unusual about the inheritance of acute intermittent porphyria?

It is an autosomal dominant disorder

Which erythropoietic porphyria is autosomal dominant inheritance?

EPP
(the one with skin lesions on exposure to light, gall stones, and mild liver dysfunction)

What is the most famous purine disorder, and how is it inherited?

- **Lesch–Nyhan**
- **X-linked**

Which enzyme is missing in Lesch–Nyhan syndrome, and why is that enzyme important?

- **HGPRT**
- **Responsible for salvaging nucleotides**

What is the presentation of a Lesch–Nyhan newborn?

Normal

For what symptomatic behavior are Lesch–Nyhan patients best known?

Self-mutilation

(*particularly of lips & fingers*)

What is often the first symptom of familial hypercholesterolemia?

Tendonitis or xanthomas of Achilles tendon
                    Or
Extensor tendons of hand

When do heterozygotes for familial hypercholesterolemia first develop symptoms?

In teens

(xanthomas or tendonitis)

When will homozygotes for familial hypercholesterolemia first present, and with what?	• **<5 years old** • **Planar xanthomas (flat orange-yellow lesions)**
If a child has a variety of first-degree relatives with significantly elevated LDL, what disorder should you suspect?	**Familial hypercholesterolemia**
If a vignette happens to mention that a child's parents have tendon xanthomas, what disorder should you suspect?	**Familial hypercholesterolemia**
Tendon xanthomas in the first decade of life & moderate hypercholesterolemia = what diagnosis?	**Sitosterolemia**
How high is the total cholesterol, usually, in familial hypercholesterolemia?	**600–1,000 mg/dL**
If a vignette tells you that a patient's LDL apoB level is high, although the regular LDL is normal, what is the diagnosis?	**Hyperapobetalipoproteinemia** Translation: High apoB protein
Familial combined hyperlipidemia has a variety of forms. Is the basic problem, though, with the receptor or the lipid production?	Lipid (VLDL) overproduction by the liver
Do familial combined hyperlipidemia patients usually develop xanthomas?	**No –** **Xanthomas are common with (isolated) familial hypercholesterolemia**
Patients with familial hypertriglyceridemia will have elevations of what lipid levels?	TGs & VLDL
What is the other name for familial hypertriglyceridemia?	Type IV Familial combined hyperlipidemia

If your patient has high TGs and high VLDLs, but also high levels of chylomicrons, what is he or she at risk for? (3)

1. Pancreatitis
2. Hyperinsulinemia
3. "Eruptive" xanthomas

If too many chylomicrons are circulating, what part of the lipid profile goes up?

Triglycerides

Deficiency of which enzyme will produce large quantities of circulating chylomicrons?

Lipoprotein lipase

A lot of circulating chylomicrons means that the body is having problems with what process?

Clearing dietary fat (lipoprotein lipase problem)

What low-tech test allows you to detect hyperchylomicronemia?

Let serum stand overnight – Thick creamy layer forms if chylomicrons are high

How does lipoprotein lipase deficiency usually present?

Colic or abdominal pain (usually before 10 years old)

If a patient has hyperchylomicrone-mia, what will the rest of the lipid panel look like?

**↑ TGs (>500 mg/dL)
↓ or normal HDL, LDL
(conversion process not working)**

Will adenylate deaminase deficiency patients have frequent symptoms of their disease?

Not necessarily –
Many are asymptomatic

Do adenylate deaminase deficiency patients have lab abnormalities on commonly obtained tests?

Sometimes ↑ CK

But

No myoglobinuria & muscle is normal on biopsy

A child with big, orange-yellow tonsils, splenomegaly, and peripheral neuropathy probably has what disorder?

Tangier disease

What is the problem in Tangier disease? (2)

1. HDL is low and abnormal

2. Cholesterol is deposited in unusual places

What is the eponymic name for abetalipoproteinemia?	Bassen–Kornzweig syndrome (Just be familiar with the name)
What, overall, is the problem in abetalipoproteinemia?	Fat can't be absorbed
What abnormalities are expected on the lipid profile of an abetalipoproteinemia patient?	• Chylomicron, VLDL, & LDL are absent • Cholesterol & TGs are low
What nutritional issue do abetalipoproteinemia patients have?	Fat malabsorption & Lack of fat-soluble vitamins (D, A, & K can be compensated for – E cannot)
What problems do abetalipoproteinemia patients suffer from? (3)	*Acanthocytosis* Pigmented retinopathy Cerebellar ataxia

Index

C.M. Houser, *Pediatric Genetics and Inborn Errors of Metabolism:*
A Practically Painless Review, DOI 10.1007/978-1-4939-0581-2,
© Springer Science+Business Media New York 2014